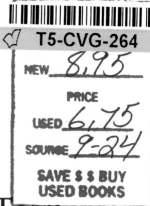

# Long-Term Care

# Care

## An Approach to Serving the Frail Elderly

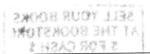

# Little, Brown Series on Gerontology

**Series Editors**

Jon Hendricks
and
Robert Kastenbaum

**Published**

Donald E. Gelfand
*Aging: The Ethnic
Factor*

Jennie Keith
*Old People
As People: Social
and Cultural
Influences on
Aging and Old Age*

Theodore H. Koff
*Long-Term Care:
An Approach
to Serving the Frail
Elderly*

**Forthcoming
Titles**

W. Andrew Achenbaum
*Aging: History
and Ideology*

Linda M. Breytspraak
*The Development
of Self in Later Life*

Carroll Estes
*Political Economy,
Health, and Aging*

Charles Harris et al.
*Applied Research
In Aging*

C. Davis Hendricks
*Law and Aging*

John L. Horn
*Aging and
Adult
Development
of Cognitive
Functions*

John F. Myles
*Political Economy
of Pensions*

Martha Storandt
*Counseling
and Psychotherapy*

Albert J.E. Wilson III
*Social Services
For Older Persons*

# Long-Term Care

## Care

### An Approach to Serving the Frail Elderly

Theodore H. Koff
University of Arizona, Tucson

Little, Brown and Company
Boston    Toronto

Library of Congress Catalog Card No.
81-86192

ISBN  0-316-500925  CB
      0-316-500933  PB

9  8  7  6  5  4  3  2  1

HAL

Published simultaneously in Canada
by Little, Brown & Company (Canada)
Limited

Printed in the United States of America

## Credits

Excerpt, pp. 105–106. From *Newer
Dimensions of Patient Care: Part I The Use of the
Physical and Social Environment of the General
Hospital for Therapeutic Purposes* by Esther Lucile
Brown, PhD. © 1961 the Russell Sage
Foundation. By permission the Russell Sage
Foundation.
Fig. 4, p. 85. From "Policies and
Strategies for Long-Term Care," Tom Joe and
Judith Meltzer, May 14, 1976. Copyright 1976
by Health Policy Program of University of
California, San Francisco (now the Institute for
Health Policy Studies, University of California,
San Francisco). Reprinted by permission.

# Contents

# Foreword
# to
# Series

Where is it? In each of the billions of cells in our bodies? Or in our minds? Then, again, perhaps it is something that happens *between* people. Ought we not also to take a look at the marketplace as well? And at the values expressed through our cultural institutions? Undoubtedly, the answer certainly lies in all of these factors—and others. The phenomenon of aging takes place within our bodies, in our minds, between ourselves and others, and as culturally defined patterns.

Burgeoning as the field is, the study and analysis of aging is deserving of an integrated spectrum approach. Now, Little, Brown offers such a perspective, one designed to respond to the diversity and complexity of the subject matter and to individualized instructional needs. The Little, Brown Series on Gerontology provides a series of succinct and readable books that encompass a wide variety of topics and concerns. Each volume, written by a highly qualified gerontologist, will provide a degree of precision and specificity not available in a general text whose coverage, expertise, and interest level cannot help but be uneven. While the scope of the gerontology series is indeed broad, individual volumes provide accurate, up-to-date presentations unmatched in the literature of gerontology.

The Little, Brown Series on Gerontology:

—provides a comprehensive overview
—explores emerging challenges and extends the frontiers of knowledge

—is organically interrelated via cross-cutting themes
—consists of individual volumes prepared by the most qualified experts
—offers maximum flexibility as teaching materials
—insures manageable length without sacrificing concepts, facts, methods, or issues.

With the Little, Brown Series on Gerontology now becoming available, instructors can select the exact mix of texts most desirable for their individual courses. Practitioners and other professionals will also find the foundations necessary to remain abreast of their own particular areas. No doubt students, too, will respond to the knowledge and enthusiasm of gerontologists writing about those topics they know and care most about.

Little, Brown and the editors are pleased to provide a series that not only looks at conceptual and theoretical questions but squarely addresses the most critical and applied concerns of the 1980s. Knowledge without action is unacceptable. The reverse is no better.

As the list of volumes makes clear, some books focus primarily on research and theoretical concerns, others on the applied; by this two-sided approach they draw upon the most significant and dependable thinking available. It is hoped that they will serve as a wellspring for developments in years to come.

# Preface

In the past, life for the long-term care provider was reasonably calm. Many of the earlier care programs were offered within the walls of an institution, with standards of care and programs reflecting the uniqueness of each institution. Payments most often were made by the resident and his or her family, with some support from the state government. I will not attempt to place a calendar date on this era of long-term care administration, preferring to call it simply the "good ole days."

But wonderful as the "good ole days" may have been, the current realities of increasing numbers of older people—especially old-old people—changing family make-up, political and economic conditions, and the state of the art require that long-term care chart a new course.

While the future of that new course is still uncertain, a whole new range of services, both institutional and noninstitutional, is envisioned. Major changes in the organization and delivery of services have occurred and will continue to evolve, especially in the area of government involvement.

Although the service requirements for people in need of long-term care have changed, caring, understanding, empathy, and competence remain essential characteristics of providers of care. It is insufficient merely to observe the dictum to do no harm. Long-term care must do good.

It is the intent of this book to help you relate the history of long-term care to a new concept in which services are developed and coordinated to respond to the ever growing needs of people living with the disabling complications of chronic illness. This is my view of what long-term care can become.

As I reminisce about the preparation of this manuscript, I wish to express a deep sense of appreciation to the many colleagues who provided valuable assistance by stimulating ideas, searching the literature, providing critical reviews, editing, and typing: Nancy Alexander, Kristine Bursac, Katherine Hoffman, Cyndi Jerald, Barbara Klijian, Marian Lupu, Deborah Monahan, Steven Rousso, Barbara Sears, Sue Shock Roderick, Dorrell-Jo MacWhinnie, and Wanda Ward.

I especially appreciate the many students who nurtured these ideas through listening, challenging, and reacting. They provided the continuing forum from which these ideas were developed.

Finally, I dedicate this book to my three children, Louis, Susan, and David, who in their dedication to me inspire my efforts to do good.

T.H.K.

# Chapter

# 1

# Introduction: What Is Long-Term Care?

The rapidly changing approaches and attitudes to care of the chronically ill reflect shifts in the issues and central concepts of the entire field of long-term care. As attitudes change, so does the terminology that describes them. Students of long-term care need both guidebook and glossary to help orient them in this rapidly changing and expanding field.

## Defining the Terms

In the early 1980s, long-term care refers to a "continuum of interrelated health and social services." It encompasses both institutional and noninstitutional services and requires coordination of public policies, funding, and case management to provide appropriate options for service to individuals whose needs inevitably change over time. Long-term care is intended to provide the individual user with choices among a variety of services, used singly or in combination, that will minimize the disabilities of chronic illness, support as independent a life-style as is practical, and prevent further complications of chronic health conditions.

Long-term care in its broadest interpretation should also encompass the education and training of providers of services, the preventive services that help avert chronic illness, and the basic research that seeks to circumvent the illnesses so often associated with the later years.

Providers and consumers of long-term care of the aging

are often uncertain of the exact meaning of such concepts as *skilled nursing care, homes for the aged, progressive care, continuum of care, extended care, campus of care, geriatric center, alternatives to institutional care, channeling agencies, case management, day care,* and so on. The proliferation of designations for various sorts of supportive institutions and agencies reflects a rush to get to too many places in too short a time. If responses to the increasing needs of an ever expanding segment of the nation's population are to be effective and economically feasible, it is essential that more order and better organization be brought to the provision of services to the elderly. Only when that has been accomplished can we hope to achieve enough unanimity about definitions within the field to be able to talk about long-term care without continual references to a glossary.

The changing names and concepts used to describe care for chronically ill older people have varied with changing systems of health delivery (e.g., *campus of care, continuum of care*), increased sophistication of the services delivered (e.g., rehabilitation and life rescue methods), the increased number of older people in society, and encompass ideas and programs from other related areas. Specific federal programs, especially those providing funds for institutional, skilled, and intermediate care, have contributed to shifting approaches and terminology. For example, concern about overexpending federal and state dollars in Medicare and Medicaid programs prompted the search for alternatives to institutional care, on the assumption that such alternatives would be less costly and therefore preferable. Thus, a new thrust in programming and research was identified and became a part of the long term care system. Programs were developed to provide new non-institutional care which met the needs of the older person adding new scope to the definition of long-term care.

Sherwood (1975) has defined a person receiving long-term care as "someone who has reached, either suddenly or gradually, a state of collapse or deterioration in human behavioral functioning which requires prolonged service from at least one other human being." These services may focus on rehabilitation, maintenance, and/or delay of further deterioration, and they include some on enhancing the quality of life.

Kaufman (1980) says that long-term care services "are geared toward helping the recipients successfully master the activities required for daily living while improving their personal satisfaction and the quality of their lives. The scope and range of this assistance is as varied as the needs of the persons served and may include such diverse services as sophisticated medical support to treat life-threatening, chronic health conditions and assistance with the daily needs of food, shelter, companionship, and supervision. Persons needing long-term care services may require care that can be defined as 'total' care or may only need assistance with those aspects of daily living that they are not able to handle for themselves."

Our understanding of what long-term care is, what it does, how it does it, and whom it serves is complicated by varieties of definitions and historical references that associated the idea of long-term care solely with institutional care. Additionally, there is what Kerschner and Cote (1979) call "deficiencies in terminology descriptive of the needs for care and services." The absence of standard nomenclature or a taxonomy of terms commonly used in long-term care results in misconceptions about the services and those to be served, and complicates the development of consistent public policies.

The definitions given below for key terms and concepts have been followed throughout the book. These definitions will clarify the long-term care continuum as it is presented here.

> *Chronic illness* refers to either physical or mental illness or to a disability caused by disease that persists over a long period of time.
>
> *Long-term care* consists of those services designed to provide diagnostic, preventive, therapeutic, rehabilitative, supportive, and maintenance services for individuals of all age groups who have chronic physical and/or mental impairments, in a variety of institutional and noninstitutional health care settings, including the home, with the goal of promoting the optimum level of physical, social, and psychological functioning.
>
> *Long-term care programs* must focus upon appropriate planning and use of all resources (medical, social, financial, rehabilitative, and supportive) needed by individuals who have continuing care needs (National Conference on Social Welfare, 1977). Services should be multidisciplinary, calling upon the resources of the related health and social services to meet the disparate needs of the chronically ill.
>
> *Continuum* is defined as a close union of related parts of a service system, including services offered at home, in nonresidential service centers, in housing programs, and in institutional facilities.
>
> A *long-term care facility* is defined to mean any skilled nursing facility or intermediate care facility as defined by the Social Security Act, sheltered or personal care or congregate care facility.
>
> *Single point of entry* refers to an organizational concept of access for any available service in the long-term care system. The single point of entry may in fact be located at any of several different physical locations such as a nursing home or social service agency. The single point of entry is the sole route of entry into the system, and therefore may be controlled to insure appropriate assessment of needs and assignment of services.

*Case Management* is a process of coordinating services for the elderly. It provides access to the entire services system and ensures the coordinated delivery of multiple services to individual clients. Basic to case management is an initial broad-based assessment of the client's needs. In addition, the case management process involves ensuring that a service plan which considers all available service solutions is written, that the client is actually connected to service, and that the progress of the client is re-examined at regular intervals.

# The Basics of a Comprehensive Care System

The Older Americans Act, especially the amendments enacted in 1978 and continued through 1981, reinforced the current emphasis on a comprehensive long-term care system and the coordination of institutional and noninstitutional services into a rational service delivery system. Title III of the amendments states its purpose as:

. . . to encourage and assist state and local agencies to concentrate resources in order to develop greater capacity and foster the development of comprehensive and coordinated services systems to serve older individuals by entering into new cooperative arrangements in each state with state and local agencies, and with the providers of social services, including nutrition services and multipurpose senior centers, for the planning for the provision of social services, nutrition services, and multipurpose senior centers, in order to

1. secure and maintain maximum independence and dignity in a home environment for older individuals capable of self-care with appropriate supportive services;
2. remove individual and social barriers to economic and personal independence for older individuals; and
3. provide a continuum of cae for the vulnerable elderly.

The act later defines a "comprehensive and coordinated system" to mean "a system for providing all necessary social services," including nutrition services, in a manner designed to:

1. facilitate accessibility to, and utilization of, all social services and nutrition services provided within the geographic area served by such system by any public or private agency or organization;
2. develop and make the most efficient use of social services and nutrition services in meeting the needs of older individuals; and
3. use available resources efficiently and with a minimum of duplications.

While comprehensive, coordinated systems of service are promoted as the goal, the coordination intended by the Older Americans Act refers to noninstitutional services, namely nutrition and social services. Yet the intent of the Act is to "provide a continuum of care for the vulnerable elderly." So while we might be positively swayed by the suggestions of comprehensiveness and coordination, the intent of the act is limited because it separates the institutional and noninstitutional portions of long-term care, and ignores vital parts of a continuum of care—namely, health care and the institutional sector.

Furthermore, since no definition of "vulnerable" is included in the act, we can only assume that programs should attempt to defend older people from the ravages of illness, the hazards of institutionalization, the trauma of dependence, and the frustration of attempting to obtain the most appropriate service in the maze of an uncoordinated health care delivery system. You have to find a dragon before you can slay it. Random, misdirected, ill-defined programs cannot be expected to help older people. It should be obvious that because the Act itself cannot respond to all of their needs, vulnerable elderly people will probably continue to be vulnerable despite legislative declarations. We find what Estes (1979) refers to as "contradictory myths" in public pronouncements: "The symbolic aspects of the goals of the Older Americans Act reassure the public that somehow the aged are being cared for, while policy is simultaneously constructed so that its material impact will not disrupt the ongoing functioning or power arrangements within society. The intentionally ambiguous language of the Older Americans Act prevents both a clear understanding of the problem and a testing of the alternatives."

Of greater consequence for long-term care services is the fact that while the Older Americans Act attempts to establish national policy, albeit confusedly, it is the administrators of Titles XVIII, XIX, and XX of the Social Security Act—not the Administration on Aging—who have access to the major sources of money for implementing programs in long-term care. Therefore, the administration on aging does not have control of the funds which could be used to implement programs it proposes. A rational planning policy should integrate the functions of planning and the provision of services while assuring that the programs designed to serve the frail elderly are appropriately funded. What remains elusive is a coherent policy theme that focuses on older people in our society rather than on the systems for delivering social service. What is lacking is the essential underpinning of a commitment by society to its elders.

An effective national program of long-term care should begin with a clear statement of what older citizens can rightfully expect from the rest of society. Without this basic understanding, older persons, their families and advocates, service providers, and society at large can neither agree on an acceptable minimum level of services nor wholeheartedly support the efforts required to enable each older person to remain a healthy, active member of society.

Good health, a positive outlook, and continued involvement in the community are in part responses to society's expressed expectations. The roles assumed by older persons reflect their society's expectations. If our society were to communicate greater approval for independence and expected good health in old age rather than accepting a developmental model that assumes gradually diminishing physical and mental capacities, growing old would be viewed very differently.

It is also important to understand clearly the differences between aging and illness, but to be aware at the same time of the relationship between increased age and the presence of some chronic illness and to recognize that older people may require additional time to recuperate from an acute illness. Aggressive treatment of disease may be as appropriate for the older person as for a young person, and is dependent upon a thorough and appropriate diagnosis. The inherent danger is that disease will be assumed to be an inevitable part of aging and, therefore, not appropriately treated. "In spite of the attention to chronic diseases and dysfunctions that accompany advancing years, aging itself—reflection of the many molecular, cellular, and systemic processes that take place with time, is not a disease" (Weg 1978). Shanas (1971) had already discussed this important idea almost ten years earlier when she said: " 'Old age' is commonly and popularly associated with illness. There seems to be general scientific agreement, however, that there is no such disease as 'old age,' and that illness is not a necessary concomitant of growing old." Appreciation of the difference between aging and illness is essential if we are to pursue aggressively the causes of illness among the elderly.

Society's response to the needs of the elderly cannot be expressed in services alone. It should begin with an acceptance of aging and the presence in our population of increasing numbers of older people. Opportunities through which increasing numbers of older persons can maintain a continuity in their life-styles and expectations should then be identified by society. It also is important to understand the social forces that cause undue stress on older individuals and create the need for substantial remedial services. Problems of changing neighborhoods, inadequate housing, limited income, and inadequate health assessment, services, or education, are among the forces that can ultimately lead to the need for long-term care—either institutional or noninstitutional. It would be more productive for society to find ways to eliminate these sources of trauma and thereby reduce the chances of prolonged illness.

# Some Cross-National Comparisons

It is helpful to compare long-term care in this country with the experiences of other developed countries. Shanas (1971) provides information about the care of the frail older person in five countries—the United States, Denmark, Great Britain, Israel, and Poland—during the late 1960s: "In every country studied some old people are residents in institutions for the elderly. Usually those in institutions are among the oldest and frailest persons in the elderly population." Additionally, Shanas reports that ". . . in each country between two and three times as many persons are bedfast and housebound in their own homes as there are in institutions of all kinds, including institutions for the well aged." Shanas summarizes her report as follows: "In each country from four to five old people in every hundred are institutionalized. From eight to fifteen in every hundred, depending on the country, are either bedfast or housebound and living in their own homes. An additional six to sixteen in every hundred are able to go outdoors only with difficulty."

These findings are echoed by Kane and Kane (1976) when they report on their study of long-term care in six countries, and the "difficulty of finding a single, all-encompassing solution for the care of the elderly. In each of the countries visited, the principal policy was to develop services that would enable the elderly to remain in their own homes, within a familiar community, for as long as possible." It was a common observation of each country that an older person—even when chronically ill—preferred to remain at home rather than enter an institution. This appears to be so even when the institution may offer greater opportunities for care and for socialization with peers. Because there are many more chronically ill people living at home than in institutions, an approach to serving the frail elderly should concentrate on helping them remain at home with appropriate services, and with access to institutional care when necessary.

Institutions have varying functions and priorities within a national long-term care plan. For example, institutional care in the United States has, in the recent past, been viewed as synonymous with long-term care. The British, on the other hand, see institutional solutions as a last resort (Kane and Kane 1976): "Under the National Health Service System, a strong hospital-based geriatric program has been developed, with an emphasis on sophisticated diagnostic assessment and supported by a strong community-based home-care program." Kane and Kane (1976) report that in other countries— namely Scotland, Norway, Israel, and the Netherlands—either a geriatric assessment unit or a nationally supported screening program determines who will be assigned to an institution or other levels of care.

In all countries reported above, a common concern has been that of rising costs accompanied by an increase in the numbers of older people requiring services. Public planners assumed that early detection of problems along with the availability of options for noninstitutional care would assist in stabilizing the national expenditures for long-term care services. This has not yet been supported by research studies in the countries studied by Kane and Kane.

A significant difference between the United States and the other countries reported is the amount of control exercised by the federal government in the provision of care to the chronically ill: "Nowhere does the profit motive figure as importantly in the arrangements for the elderly as it does in the United States . . ." (Kane and Kane 1976). Yet in the other countries, far more control was placed in the hands of local authorities than is the case in the United States. There seems to be some correlation, although unmeasured, between the role of the national government, the responsibility of local governments, and governmental support of institutional care (Kane and Kane 1976). While few conclusions can be drawn from these observations, it does become apparent that efforts to develop a comprehensive long-term care program in this country will have to deal with some of the same policy issues confronted by other countries.

Most countries studied by Kane and Kane had identified problems in the separation of the health and social care systems for the elderly, and, subsequently, the nature of the linkages between them. We see the same disparity in Titles XVIII, XIX, and XX of the Social Security Act, where strong emphasis on medical care in nursing homes contrasts with a focus on social aspects of long-term care outside the institution. The disparity also appears in various health and social welfare jurisdictions at the federal and state government levels.

Another area in which the United States differs from other countries is in the recognition of geriatric medicine as a specialty supported by departments of geriatrics in medical schools. Anderson (1979) identifies Italy, Spain, England, Australia, and New Zealand as countries that recognize geriatrics as a subspecialty of general medicine and have endowed Chairs in geriatrics in their medical schools. In contrast, the Institute of Medicine (1978) in the United States recommends that geriatrics be integrated into appropriate areas of medical education and practice rather than being supported as a subspecialty. The documented problems of physicians caring for older persons in nursing homes (Miller, Lowenstein, and Winston 1976; Kane and Kane 1980b), and the limited programs in geriatric medicine in this country's medical schools (Kane and Kane 1980) indicate that hesitancy to move forthrightly into a geriatric specialty may be evidence of an absence of commitment to geriatric medicine. Establishing medical specialization is not in itself a resounding response to the needs of older persons, but it could represent a partial acknowledgement that geriatric medicine is an essential component of better care to the chronically ill elderly.

A common theme in the literature of foreign countries, and one that is of great concern in this country, is the role of the family in providing care for the frail elderly, either in a common residence or in separate households. Bengtson (1979), discussing this theme, says that in the United States:

> The changing family context of older people is the source of considerable concern on the part of many lay persons and practitioners. Examination of the available research in terms of the five constructs of solidarity, however, reveals many beliefs about contemporary family life to be false. For example, despite dramatic changes in demographic composition (and thus family structure), most older individuals appear to have high rates of interaction with children, regard the intergenerational relationship as warm and close, and exchange a great deal of assistance and support. Service bureaucracies appear not to supplant, but rather supplement, the family in providing needed services.

Delegates to the 1980 White House Conference on Families urged that tax incentives be established both to make it easier for households with elderly members to remain intact and, when necessary, to modify the home to accommodate the needs of older people. Delegates recognized that younger families caring for elderly relative often could cope better if services directed to implementing appropriate care were available.

Yet the maintenance of close family bonds may in some cases result from an inadequate welfare program that is supposed to provide services to the elderly, or a national government so committed to other national priorities that it is unable to assume greater responsibility for the elderly (Bergman 1979; Yamamuro 1979). Bergman further adds that: "The belief that the aged are respected and provided for by these families and/or self-sufficient continues all too often to serve as justification for a lack of action." The interaction of aging individuals with their families was the theme of The Gerontological Society of America's 1980 Annual Scientific Meeting, which brought into sharp focus the importance of the family to each individual. In long-term care, the family may hold the key to issues of cost control, the feasibility of an individual's remaining at home, and the quality of care obtained from service agencies. For example, a family in which all adult members are employed may find it difficult to provide care to a dependent parent. A family member monitoring the care given to their parent may promote the quality and continuity of that care.

Chronically ill older persons, by the nature of the problems of chronic illness, are incapable of massing an advocacy effort on their own behalf. The absence of such advocacy or concerned interest groups leaves the frail elderly inadequately represented in the process of developing public policies in this country. While an advocacy role has to some extent been assumed by care providers, such representation lacks the strong human interest element so central in other successful advocacy efforts. In the absence of a more coherent public policy, each family's resourcefulness may well determine the quality of basic care and social support an older person receives.

## Summary

The current status of long-term care is an outgrowth of historical events in health and social service programs specifically related to the elderly, funding programs, and technological advances in health care, as well as current politics and public policies. An examination of experiences in other developed countries sheds light on some common factors cutting across national boundaries. These include the role of the family, the increasing cost for services, increases in the numbers of chronically ill individuals, the preference of older people to remain at home but still be able to receive needed services, separation or integration of social and health care systems, and concern for the increasing numbers of chronically mentally impaired people needing support.

In the United States we have experienced many of the same problems and tried or considered some similar programs. But, perhaps because of our geographic size, we have not been able to integrate national policies or services for those who are chronically ill. Much more needs to be learned and implemented. At least we know that, by itself, offering services has not resolved the problem. Cross-national studies give further impetus to the need for research into the causes, prevention, and treatment of chronic illness, public policies designed to respond to the problems, and the reshaping of programs to be more responsive to pressing needs. It is against this background that this book will discuss new approaches to serving the frail elderly in the context of long-term care.

# Chapter

# 2

# Long-Term Care: Its Emergence and Development

*The philosophy of Medicare emphasizes health care for acute illness over other needs. The aged population certainly suffers from acute illnesses, but their major health difficulties are largely chronic and often relate to a decline in their functional capacity, their ability to care for themselves in everyday situations. Yet these long-term care problems are not given the priority of acute or short-term, hospital-based emergencies. In our conscientious desire to preserve life we have ignored the needs of the living.*

CARL EISDORFER

Long-term care, as a framework for responding to the needs of chronically ill older people, should: (1) generate funds and services to assist older people who have chronic impairments, to overcome the limitations of the impairment; (2) develop the policies, resources, and services that will prevent some of the problems related to chronic illness; and (3) take into account the aspects of our society that make the older person vulnerable to chronic illness.

Long-term care services should be viewed as society's committed response to the needs of older persons beset by the disabilities of chronic illness, which are complicated and aggravated by inadequate responses from the social, medical, educational, familial, and spiritual resources of the community. It is not enough to think of long-term care as neatly divided into institutional and noninstitutional services, to examine alternatives to any existing services, or to concentrate on developing new ways to encourage cooperation among federal or other service agencies. "Discussions of long-term care alternatives tend to resemble cacophony more than a symphony. In addition to confusion over different meanings of alternatives other social themes are discordantly interspersed. There is no consensus on the reasons for the pursuit of alternatives . . ." (Kane and Kane 1980a).

A societal commitment to chronically ill elderly should be expressed as a national policy. Public adoption of such a policy should then be followed by strong support for the research necessary to build the knowledge base on which an effective delivery system can be developed for relevant services as well as preventive programs. The stated public commitment would provide a baseline against which accomplishments in long term-care could be evaluated. Public commitment also provides a support base for the allocation of the funds necessary to carry out the long-term care programs.

## Family Support Systems

At the same time the problems of long-term care are being approached from the macrolevel of public policy and major community commitments, it is essential that family and community support systems on behalf of the frail elderly be strengthened, since these are the essential foundation for any long-term care system. Shanas (1979b) argues that it is a myth "that in contemporary American society old people are alienated from their families, particularly from their children." Acknowledgement of this observation can become the basis of a support structure that takes advantage of the existing family network. "Further," Shanas continues, "where old people have no children, a principle of family substitution seems to operate and brothers, sisters, nephews, and nieces often fulfill the roles and assume the obligations of children. The truly isolated old person, despite his or her prominence in the media, is a rarity in the United States."

In a 1968 study Shanas found that families regularly perform household tasks for their older relatives and often house their relatives with them in times of crisis. Townsend (1965) found that older persons frequently moved in with their families until severe circumstances forced their institutionalization. York and Calsyn (1977) reaffirmed these earlier studies indicating that families do not separate themselves from their older relatives until they perceive themselves as no longer capable of providing the needed care. York and Calsyn found, however, that when an older person is referred to a nursing home following hospitalization, families often are not thorough in their search for a nursing home or for those services that might have enabled the older person to return home after the period of hospitalization. At the time of their study, communities may not have had the comprehensive services that would have made a direct return home possible. Care providers may not then have had the knowledge of methods by which institutionalization could have been avoided when appropriate home care services were available. Because family involvement in any decision related to a program of long-term care for relatives is vital, Shanas (1979b) says, we must stop treating families as if they were "enemies of the system."

While organizations in our society have replaced many of the support functions expected from families, "It is still the family, that group of individuals related by blood or marriage, that is the first resource of both its older and younger members for emotional and social support, crisis intervention, and bureaucratic linkages" (Shanas 1979b). Yet is it wrong to assume that supportive, willing, and loving families will have the competence or capacity to provide continuous care for chronically ill older people no longer capable of functioning without ongoing support.

"In all developed countries, as individual needs both increase and are differently defined, functions which may once have been the unique province of the family become shared functions of the family and bureaucracy, whether the latter be government, industry, or the educational system" (Shanas 1979a). The importance of the role of the family in response to the call for help from family members is supported by findings from many countries: "Research evidence indicates that family help, particularly in time of illness, exchange of services, and regular visits are common among old people and their children and relatives whether or not these live under a single roof. Old people living under a single roof together with their children and grandchildren are unusual in industrialized societies and are becoming less common in transitional societies. Joint living is not the most important factor governing the relationship between old people and their grown children. Rather, it is the emotional bond between parents and children that is of primary importance" (Shanas 1979a).

Brody, Poulshock, and Masciocchi (1978), in a study to "identify the variables which govern the institutional or community placement of the functionally disabled older person," discovered that the critical variable was the person's living arrangement. Such a person living with spouse and/or children was most likely to remain at home. Individuals with similar levels of impairment as those who were institutionalized lived at home because of the presence of a family member. Dunlop (1980) reports similar findings: "Those experiencing the lowest use of nursing homes were the ones who had another household member available to provide informal care." Dunlop then asks, "If this indeed is the case, how many families could be encouraged, through expansion of home-based services, to care for dependent elderly members any longer than they already do, or to care for very sick relatives who require continuous care?"

In a study of a group of older persons in Great Britain, 42 percent of the respondents received some form of help from visiting relatives. While this figure supports the observation that families do provide resources to the older person, "The danger remains that because this argument is substantially valid, it is used to obscure the crisis situations currently experienced by a growing minority of older people whose needs for care far exceed the capabilities of ordinary families in their own homes—or who simply do not have any supporting relatives" (Pinker 1980). Pinker further discusses the family's relationship to problems of chronic illness in Great Britain, saying, ". . . it can no longer be assumed that the families of the very aged, an increasing proportion of whom will be mentally infirm, incontinent, or terminally ill, will have the willingness and the capacity to give them the necessary care and support in their own homes, for as much as ten years or more."

The same problem of the changing function of the family in long-term care is noted by Grunow (1980) in West Germany, as he cites the decrease in family size that has resulted in fewer three-generation families, more two-generation households, and increasing numbers of "elderly single women living alone and apart from their children." Grunow also reports that "elderly and their children do wish to live in separate households rather than in the same household."

In Japan, the majority of the aged still live with their relatives and it is not expected that this custom will change drastically in the future (Okazaki 1979). However, Yamamuro (1979) reports that the number of older people living independently has risen from 3.6 percent in 1960 to 6.8 percent in 1975. This has caused alarm in a society committed to maintaining the customs of the extended family. In 1975, 76 percent of those over sixty-five continued to live with married children, compared with about 30 percent in the United States and Europe.

Shanas's contention that the alienation of old people from their families is primarily a myth is further supported by evidence that families continue to provide the bulk of the care received by older people in the United States (U.S. Dept. HEW National Center for Health Statistics 1972). A full appreciation of the role of the family in providing support is important as we look to ways of strengthening services provided for chronically ill older people.

## The Impact of Demographic Changes on Family and Long-Term Care

In 1978, 24.1 million people in the United States, or one person in every nine, was sixty-five years of age or older. Between 1900 and 1978, the percentage of the U.S. population aged sixty-five or over more than doubled, from 4.1 percent in 1900 to 11.0 percent in 1978, while the numbers increased eight times (from 3 million to 24 million). At present death rates, the older population is expected to increase an additional 32 percent to 32 million by the year 2000. If the present low birth rate persists, these 32 million will be 12.2 percent of the total population of about 260 million (Facts About Older Americans 1979).

"The single demographic change that is bound to have one of the most profound and far-reaching effects on the family, and through it eventually on society at large, is the increase in the number and proportion of the old old population" (Lipman 1979). Neugarten (1974), differentiating needs of older persons according to age, designated those people aged fifty-five to seventy-five as the "young old" and those over seventy-five as the "old old." "This division recognizes that those aged fifty-five to seventy-five are generally able to maintain themselves in most respects without assistance; they retain functional independence. Those aged seventy-five and over, although desirous of achieving autonomy, independence, and self-sufficiency, require much more aid to enable them to cope with the demands of everyday life and to complete their lives in the freedom and privacy of their own dwellings (Lipman 1979). Brotman (1978) points out that more than two million Americans are eighty-five years of age or older, and that it is these numbers and the numbers of those moving into this category that represent a major concern in long-term care.

For example, in 1977 there were 18,300 nursing homes, with 1,383,600 beds which served 1,297,400 residents (U.S. Dept. HEW National Center for Health Statistics 1978). "Almost 90 percent of those in nursing homes were sixty-five and over, and the median age was about eighty-two. Since the median age of all people in the United States aged sixty-five and over is seventy-three, it is obvious that the chance of admission to an institution increases with advancing age. In fact, only 2 percent of the sixty-five to seventy-four group, but about 10 percent of those eighty and over, are institutionalized. Of the institutionalized elderly, about 17 percent are sixty-five to seventy-four, 40 percent are seventy-five to eighty-four, and 43 percent are eighty-five and older. The fact that the seventy-five and over group is growing at a much more rapid rate than the sixty-five to seventy-four group indicates that the proportion of the very old in institutions will increase" (Brody 1977).

The impact of the aging of our society is also seen in the incidence of nursing home use. Persons sixty-five to seventy-four spent an average of 4.4 days per year in a nursing home in 1974. This increased to 21.5 days for the seventy-five to eighty-four-year-old group and rose to 86.4 days for those eighty-five years of age and older. Chronic illnesses are more prevalent among older persons than younger. In 1977, about 37 percent of older people were limited in their major activity (working or keeping house) due to such conditions, as compared to only 7 percent for younger persons (Facts About Older Americans 1979).

Lipman (1979) notes that the most significant characteristics of persons aged seventy-five and over related to the concerns of long-term care are: "(a) they are more likely to be socially isolated as measured by their living alone and widowhood; (b) they have fewer financial resources, lower income, and assets; (c) they are substantially limited in physical performance; (d) they demonstrate an increase in chronic illness as well as functional decline; (e) they utilize health services at a higher rate; (f) their rate of institutionalization is higher; (g) they are more likely to have children who are themselves approaching old age, or are old."

The increase in numbers of the old old population, along with the reduction of the number of descendants, or what Lipman (1979) calls the "thinning out of the kinship network," has set the stage for new developments in long-term care services. "The family is the primary support system of the elderly person residing in the community with some degree of independence. It is also the primary resource in maintaining the aged in the community in the face of chronic illness and functional decline." Approaches used to develop long-term care services should first seek ways to buttress the family and its competence and capacity to cope with the increasing demands and strains, then augment the family resources with community services that permit the family to maintain its supportive involvement.

Rakowski and Hickey (1980) suggest that "older adults may possess constricted future expectations. More specifically, individuals may evidence less distant personal projection, fewer expected life events, and/or perceive a less important future. Other factors which may reflect change are in the direction of less future planning and a future of less anticipated pleasantness." This temporal dimension, or the absence of belief that the future is important, is certain to have some impact on the health behavior of older people. The potential for family involvement in caring for the chronically ill older person may be enhanced by the family's ability to support a positive future image for the older person. This in turn may strengthen the family's commitment to the future of the older person, as well as prove supportive to the family members who later are able to transfer the more positive temporal aspects to their own aging and self-image.

There seems to be an important difference between the reaching out of the older person for family support and the subsequent response of the family to ask for help from community service agencies. Often, when the family is called upon to assist the older person who may be in distress, the family responds by calling on the community services or care provider rather than providing the service. This is especially true when family members no longer live in the same household as their elders.

When a family reaches out for help, its members may not adequately understand either the needs of their relative or the resources of varied health and social services in the community. They may therefore seek only sources with which they have already become familiar, or may avoid other resources on the basis of vague negative impressions. Services chosen in this manner may not be appropriate. Avoiding inappropriate service—that which is inadequate or more intensive than is required—is one of the goals of the coordinated approach to long-term care. Past attempts to evolve a long-term care system have focused on postponing the time when the family must search for help from supportive services or on directing the individual or family to an appropriate case management or facilitator service that will introduce the family to the services available within the long-term care system. Entry into a system of long-term care can be most beneficial when it provides an appropriate assessment of both the individual's and the family's needs and strengths, followed by involvement in the appropriate elements of the system that will provide the services that are required. These elements include family supports such as education and counseling in addition to the services provided for the chronically ill person.

Smith and Bengtson (1979) found that institutionalization of the chronically ill relative strengthens family relations with renewed and continued closeness. This probably results from the reduced stress on the family once the ill member is removed.

Perhaps a more productive entry into the long-term care system would begin with a case manager working with the family, including the older person. Counselors and families must become more adept in finding a suitable entry point into the long-term care system for the person in need in addition to providing direct service.

Long-term care obviously includes more than institutional care or the combination of institutional and noninstitutional services. Long-term care should include preventive and educational services as well as the full gamut of health and social services, organized and controlled through case management with adequate funding to support all of these services. This approach appears to be consistent with the 1978 Amendments' to the Older Americans Act recommendations for comprehensive and coordinated service systems and a continuum of care for vulnerable elderly people.

## Alternatives to Institutional Care

In the early 1970s, attention focused on the issue of "alternatives" to institutional care. This was an understandable reaction to exposés of poor programs and evidence of overcharging. There was concern about the increasing number of institutional beds being occupied for long-term care, and the subsequent increasing proportion of the national health care budget spent on institutional long-term care.

Kaplan (1972) succinctly summarized the issues by challenging some of the following underlying assumptions:

> First, there are alternatives.
> Next, nursing home care is the last stop.
> Further, independent home care is better for the aged American than nursing home care.
> People prefer to remain in their own homes under all conditions.
> Home care is cheaper than nursing home care, and many people do not have to be in nursing homes.

Kaplan argues that "choices" may have been a better selection of words for the discussion than "alternatives": "Choices indicate an armamentarium of services which will allow for the proper service selection. Alternatives indicate that other service types could replace the nursing home. The aim should be to keep people from being underserviced, overserviced, or misserviced, not to give a negative connotation to nursing home or institutional care based on the lowest level of such care offered." He further argued that what was needed were parallel systems of institutional care with a method for cross-integrating the two. The goal, Kaplan stated, is to have "a complete range of choices through a continuum of services."

Other theorists promoted the ideal of a constellation of services, an assemblage of all the required parts for a total program; or a continuum of services, an unbroken link of related services. Bell (1973) defined the concept of community care as including those noninstitutional services which may prevent or delay premature institutionalization. Community care would coordinate five basic home-delivered services offered through a single public agency: (1) health maintenance; (2) help with housekeeping and shopping; (3) meals; (4) transportation to health and essential services; and (5) counseling, crisis intervention, and advocacy. Furthermore, "a comprehensive long term program of health care should satisfy at least these criteria: quality, accessibility, acceptability, equity, flexibility, centralized responsibility, and accountability."

While one could hardly find fault with these criteria, presentations of the concept of alternatives have sometimes implied that community care and institutional care are mutually exclusive. Such a presentation denies the essence of those criteria. Criticizing institutional care in order to emphasize the value of home care is not productive since the two are complementary. Accessibility, acceptability, equity, and centralized responsibility and accountability require a unification of institutional and noninstitutional modes of care into a comprehensive system of care, without competition between them to determine which level of care is to be preferred.

The validity of an estimate that as many as 5 percent or more of the older population are in nursing homes (Kastenbaum and Candy 1973) was widely disputed in the early 1970s. Kastenbaum and Candy challenged the figures as an inappropriate use of cross-sectional data: "Knowing how many elders are institutionalized at this moment, no matter how accurate a statement, does not tell us how many people will have resided in extended care facilities at some time in their lives." Their study found that one of four older persons died in an extended care facility, suggesting a figure far in excess of 5 percent: "The misleading usage of extended care facility population statistics tends to draw attention away from the fact that many of our elders end their lives among strangers in an environment that offers little 'nursing' and scarcely resembles a 'home.' " More positively, the authors say that "every action that is taken to improve the quality of life in extended care facilities will be a blessing to a very considerable number of our fellow citizens." We cannot misuse the 5 percent figure to suggest that institutional care is an insignificant portion of the total long-term care system. It is, in fact, a very substantial part of the service, and attracts a significant proportion of the money available for all long-term care services.

An analogous concern regarding statistics on long-term care was raised by Kisten and Morris (1972) on the issue of inappropriate placement in an institutional setting because of the absence of basic supportive services in the home. In a subsequent paper, Morris (1974) estimated that anywhere between 15 percent and 40 percent of the populations of proprietary nursing homes could benefit from home care in lieu of the institutionalization. Morris finds fault with what he refers to as "existing arteriosclerotic financial arrangements which give a privileged position to institutional care in contrast with alternative modalities." Service providers and families alike find it easier to obtain necessary services on an ongoing basis through institutionalization rather than through home care because of the funding priority given to institutional care by the third party payers.

In 1962, Shanas (1971) found that "there seems to be a hard core of bedfast and housebound elderly ranging between 8 percent and 14 percent of the total elderly population." She later found, in a 1975 survey, that this percentage had not changed markedly since 1962, suggesting that despite all the advances in health care financing programs of the late 1960s, there were no changes in the proportion of institutionalized and homebound aged. The Shanas survey also found that the "greatly impaired are most likely to be in institutions and less impaired are most likely still to be at home." These findings helped place in perspective the importance of providing home care for those who were homebound and not involved in institutional care.

Shore suggested in 1974 that the new issues in the discussions of alternatives were, "first, the possibility of payments for parallel services, and second, the recognition that isolated scattered, freestanding, helter-skelter alternatives will not work. A coordinated program of institutional and parallel services—a supermarket of services is required."

He advocated that our concern should be not for the 5 percent institutionalized population, nor any other segment, but rather should be directed at 100 percent of the elderly population. "The institution should be thought of as one link in the chain of services—not the weakest link, or the sickest, least desirable link, or the final link; simply another link." The most important part of his thesis is his advocacy of health care of the elderly as a right rather than a privilege. Accepting this assumption permits the enlargement of the conceptual delivery system to include a much broader variety of services.

Fears that the absence of a comprehensive approach to the needs of the frail elderly will contribute to a rapid increase in institutionalization because it is the most accessible service response may be justified. Attempts to coordinate services and to increase resources cannot by themselves allay these fears. Before the concept of a true continuum of care can be widely and enthusiastically accepted, there must be both a better understanding of what services will be most beneficial to the chronically ill and a major reexamination of priorities by various segments of government which share responsibilities for chronically impaired older people (Estes 1979).

The goal of maintaining older persons in their own households is not appropriate for those individuals whose health and social needs may be denied through this support of independence. In essence, people can be inappropriately institutionalized within their own households if remaining there deprives them of access to the services generally offered in an institutional environment. A dichotomy between institutional and noninstitutional service is not the crux of the problem. Until we approach the problems of chronically impaired older people with a more precise understanding of how best to match their needs with the services that should be provided to meet them, we cannot hope to communicate those needs and proposed responses to various levels of government in a manner that will inspire a firm commitment of the necessary funds.

To a large extent, we don't know how best to respond to the problems of the large number of chronically impaired older people among us because the problem is relatively new to government and service providers alike. The problem is made more difficult because service providers generally give low priority to caring for chronically ill elderly people. Such people are not expected to become productive, and productivity is a highly valued goal in our society. In addition, the large numbers of the client group combine with the high cost of care of chronic conditions to project a gloomy outlook.

## Long-Term Care As a Concept

How then should we consider long-term care? Should it be defined as a prolonged institutionalization in contrast to a short term stay in an acute care hospital? Standard health care terminology that frequently pairs acute care and long-term care compares the *nature* of illness (acute) with a period of time (long-term). To be analogous, the fields should be defined either by levels of illness or by length of stay (i.e., acute or chronic; short-term or long-term). Possibly a better term for long-term care might be chronic care, and some criteria could be established that would distinguish it from acute care. There are other considerations. Acute care generally refers to care provided within the hospital, or acute-care setting. Long-term care or chronic care, in contrast, is more often provided outside an institution than within. To be accurate, the definition of chronic care should avoid treating it as synonymous with institutionalization and measuring it solely in terms of length of stay.

An approach to developing a definition of long-term care is provided by Brody (1977), who describes long-term care as "one or more services provided on a sustained basis to enable individuals whose functional capacities are chronically impaired to be maintained at their maximum levels of health and well being." She also says that "relevant issues are to identify those for whom long-term care is appropriate and to determine the nature of the services and the qualities of the environments that would maximize their well-being."

In our current services for the chronically ill it is recognized that "appropriateness" of home care or institutional care should be a major criterion for selecting services that will augment well being. The observation that a segment of the institutional population may be inappropriately institutionalized often suggests that although members of this group could have been cared for outside the institution, realities of our society encourage institutionalization. For example, it is still easier to obtain payments for institutional care on a prolonged basis than it is to obtain the same support for noninstitutional care. Health care providers have been reluctant to offer close supervision for those living at home alone, and have instead encouraged institutionalization whenever there has been a question about the availability or quality of supports at home. Institutionalization has often been viewed as a permanent transfer of residence, prompting the disposal of prior residences and household furnishings, thus making it impossible for the person to return to his or her own home.

In addition to the pressures for institutionalization produced by funding of service providers, institutions have been advocates for their own use, especially when vacancies exist. Administrators often display anxiety when occupancy is low and respond to this anxiety by marketing institutional care to the service providers, physicians, social agencies, and hospitals. The administrative goal is clearly that of maintaining high occupancy, which is understandable since budgets and payments for nursing home care are determined by the level of occupancy. It would be administratively irresponsible to treat the issue of low occupancy casually. Furthermore, low occupancy generally results in lower quality of care for those residing in the institution because the ability to maintain services is dependent upon a high level of income, which in turn is usually dependent upon high occupancy. Institutions are not rewarded for vacancies that might occur if new applicants were accepted only after a most thorough search of ways to care for the person at home. Similarly, institutions are inclined to accept patients on the basis of the needs of the administration—namely, the desire to have a patient mix which requires a combination of heavy and light care, or of patients for whom it is more or less costly to provide care. If those persons who were "inappropriately" placed in nursing homes were transferred out, or were directed to noninstitutional programs, the resultant institutional population would be increasingly more frail and dependent and the per capita cost of providing appropriate care would rise. Patients who would be discharged from nursing homes would tend to be "the minimal care cases—those independently ambulating, continent, and mentally clear" (Davis and Gibbons 1971). There is no assurance that the residual institutional population demanding greater care would command a higher per diem reimbursement.

It must therefore be recognized that noninstitutional programs that could successfully reduce the institutionalization of minimal care cases might have immediate impact on the institutional case load, demands on staff, institutional program, and services that would lead to increased costs for institutional care (Davis and Gibbons 1971). These anticipated effects will obviously provoke some resistance to reduced institutionalization.

On the acute care side of the continuum, we know that a community's experience with hospital bed use has a bearing on institutional long-term care. Where hospital beds are underused, there is less pressure to transfer patients to nursing homes. Conversely, where there is urgent need for hospital beds, patients are sometimes rushed out of the hospital without adequate time having been taken to assess the appropriate next level of care. Where there is a shortage of nursing home beds in a community, many older people are retained in the hospital for long periods awaiting nursing home placement (Rossman 1973). These circumstances highlight the importance of planning for long-term care in the context of existing and planned resources for acute care.

## Assessment of Needs

Anderson (1979) has said: "If geriatric medicine has to be summed up in one word it would be the word diagnosis." *Diagnosis* is the definition from symptoms of the true nature of an individual's problems. *Assessment* is the determination of the amount of functional limitation that can be expected from the diagnosis, and should also include an evaluation of individual capacities as well as family resources and their capacities. The health status and living situations of older people are assessed in health care practitioners' offices, hospitals, or health care centers, as well as in the home. Older people whose needs for long-term care services are assessed in an acute care facility will be seen either in an acute phase of an episode or in the sick role, wearing hospital clothes, and behaving as a hospitalized patient. This is hardly the environment in which an accurate judgment can be made regarding the patient's ability to function at home with or without home care supportive services.

Kleh (1977) recommends the use of a "geriatric evaluation unit" to study the patient's service needs and produce multidisciplinary diagnosis and treatment recommendations, providing comprehensive workups not otherwise available to the family physician. "Comprehensive evaluations ... help correct medical misconceptions about the elderly that promote premature or unnecessary institutionalization." The evaluation process should take into consideration the person's physical, psychological, and social needs and capacities. "The better the fit between the individual and the level of services received, the more likely it is that the desired patient outcomes will be achieved" (Sherwood, Morris, and Barnhart 1975).

We need also to consider the impact of the "three-day hospitalization before nursing home" Medicare requirement to qualify a patient for nursing home payments. This unquestionably promotes arbitrary and often unnecessary hospital stays, and adds to the frequency of relocation for older persons as they are transferred from the hospital to a nursing home. The relocation may be anxiety-provoking, disorienting, and, under the most adverse situations, life-threatening. Additionally, selection of the hospital as the most desirable environment in which to assess the total needs of the individual and make some judgment about subsequent nursing home placements should be questioned. The artificiality of this requirement imposes constraints on the evolving long-term care system, and should be abandoned in favor of a more reasonable approach: developing appropriate long-term care assessment centers, available on a noninstitutional basis but coordinated with inpatient facilities when necessary.

Of primary importance in the development of long-term care assessment centers is the design of an appropriate schedule for classifying patients in terms of service needs. Some who are nursing home candidates are bedridden, some are ambulatory, and some are both at different times. Yet all may have the same disease. A disease may be a precipitating factor in the decision to institutionalize a patient, but the significant consideration is how well the patient can function in the context not only of this disease or diseases but in terms of all factors that contribute to disability, including psychosocial circumstances.

The findings of one assessment study of older people both in and out of nursing homes indicate that "individuals lacking strong social and financial supports are likely to be prematurely admitted to a nursing home; thus, a socioeconomic need is met with a health care solution" (Barney 1977). An additional finding of the study is "that the strongest dynamic now at work in our society to prevent overuse of institutions is not the concern of taxpayers over unwisely spent health care dollars, not the concern of the public over the mistreatment of the elderly, but the stubborn determination of older people themselves to make it on their own. In view of this often unrecognized fact, it is up to policymakers to devise ways to place within reach of all elderly citizens the kind of help that augments self-reliance and enables them to keep their own coping systems going" (Barney 1977). This observation will often be overlooked unless the resources of an assessment center are made available to older people; it especially is obscured if the assessment process principally looks for deficits and not for strengths and capacities.

An illustration of an assessment program that enables the individual to remain at home is a program known as "aftercare," that initially was used for services to patients after hospitalization. Hospital services are provided during a daytime period for a group of about six people. The group is treated as a social group during the hospital visit, with social activities and meal(s) provided while assessment activities are performed (Rossman 1977).

The development of comprehensive assessment programs that are founded in medical, psychological, and social diagnosis is the essential backdrop for long-term care programs. While several communities in the United States have developed assessment programs, such programs have not yet become the typical point of entry into a service system. Because the Veteran's Administration is deeply committed to serve a large group of elderly veterans with chronic illnesses, that agency has pioneered in the development of geriatric assessment units at its medical centers.

Other countries, having had more experience with the delivery of long-term care services due to the earlier aging of a society in existence longer than the United States, depend more upon the use of assessment centers to determine need and admit individuals into the care network. For example, in Great Britain and Holland, all applicants for long-term care must be seen at an assessment center (Anderson 1979). In Israel and Australia, assessment centers are used in some communities to determine the appropriate level of care (Gibson 1979; Kane and Kane 1976). Assessment centers offer a setting in which to perform comprehensive diagnostic examinations, to assign services based on demonstrated need, and to avoid inappropriate use of services. Assessment centers and their use in a coordinated system represent one way to assure the most appropriate use of funds available to provide long-term care services.

# The Role of the Health Systems Agency and Licensing Issues

The local Health Systems Agency (HSA) has a significant role to play in shaping the character of long-term care. This health planning structure was created by the National Health Planning and Resource Development Act of 1974. Its establishment set the stage for development of the certificate of need process for local community review and approval of licensed health care facilities and services. The "certificate of need" is the end product of a community planning process that recommends or disapproves the addition or deletion of identified facilities or services. The denial of the request for a certificate of need generally implies that the program will not be licensed by the state, and thereby will be prohibited from offering the service.

While the HSA can encourage the start-up of new, needed services, its primary activities to date have been aimed at preventing duplication of existing services and limiting the increasing costs of health care. Given this goal of restricting growth, the HSA's have generally not been the promoters of new services. Much of what the HSA's do in projecting future needs is based retrospectively on the community's experiences, even though these may be shown to be inappropriate precedents for future service delivery to older people. For example, judgment about the need for long-term care institutional beds is based in part on experiences of past years, when related home care or day care services which might reduce the need for institutional beds, might not have been available.

Human (1976) differentiates between *forecasting,* making valid probabilistic statements about the future; and *normative planning,* the process of attempting to set and achieve ideal future goals. He argues that a planning decision based on a forecast alone ignores the values implicit in nearly any resource allocation. In the present period of developing varied institutional and noninstitutional programs, "planning for this sector should involve more than describing the present system, forecasting demand, and allocating resources to continue the system. . . . The normative health systems plan should recognize that long-term care differs from other modes of health care in that while it is ordinarily conceived of as a medical care system, it is also more of a social system for its patients. Patients are ordinarily elderly and suffering from chronic disabilities of illness that often persist for years" (Human 1976).

It is very possible that the growing public distaste for regulations and controls in all aspects of government will result in reduction of the authority of the Health Systems Agency, making it even more important that local communities develop coordinated systems of long-term care based on a network of local services rather than one that is required by federal regulations. The absence of some responsible planning procedure will perpetuate inappropriate service accompanied by inappropriate allocation of resources, and will inhibit development of a full network of long-term care services.

The continuum of long-term care services that includes institutional and noninstitutional services does not have its licensing requirements or regulations coordinated at the state level. Each program is licensed separately (wherever licensing is applicable), but there is no comprehensive license that makes it possible to incorporate multiple levels of institutional and noninstitutional care. This problem became evident when efforts were being made by hospice programs—which include a continuum of home care, institutional care, and bereavement care—to obtain a comprehensive hospice license issued under the authority of a hospice law that will include all three levels of care (Koff 1980). Hospice care is a new coordinated program to provide palliative care to patients with terminal illness, and is most effective when home care, institutional care, and day care are coordinated to permit a single point of entry and shared staff. In a like manner, long-term care that coordinates several levels of institutional and noninstitutional care needs to be treated as a continuum of coordinated services in the planning and licensing process. This, of course, is related to the procedures of the HSA, which certifies at the local level the need for a proposed service. To a large extent, judgment regarding the need for new services is based on the local health plan, developed by the HSA, that lays out the perspective of community health services. For the most part, these plans do not view an integrated continuum of care as a community goal. They also treat institutional services as separate from noninstitutional services and offer few incentives for achieving a coordinated system.

## Who Is to Lead?

Who, then, can provide the impetus to create a coordinated system of care? For the most part, stimulus has come from the Administration on Aging, through its model projects, which in turn have encouraged local communities to search for new ways to respond to the needs of an ever increasing segment of society. Model or demonstration projects have sought ways to assure greater access to existing services, to develop new services, and to assure that the older person in need can find the appropriate level of care when it is needed. Underlying all these approaches has been the important goal of conserving limited financial resources and assuring that money spent will pay for an appropriate response to the needs of the individual served.

Public agencies, i.e., state health departments, that oversee the performance of long-term care organizations, often have organizational structures that deal separately with the institutional and noninstitutional aspects of the service and with funding and licensing. It seems reasonable to suggest that agencies that either fund, license, supervise, and/or approve certificates of need in an environment where no continuum of care currently exists would have difficulty coordinating their various activities. The goals of the continuum of long-term care and services for the chronically ill have to be adopted even without prior community experiences in these areas, and despite a confused history.

There is a real need for an advocacy position that:

1. supports the premise that a continuum of long-term care is desirable for the older person, the service agencies, and the society at large;
2. requires that the elements of a continuum be written into funding patterns, regulations, and licensing procedures;
3. assures coordination of the approval of services and the allocation of money to support the use of the service; it is untenable that the Health Systems Agency can approve the development of a new service without the concomitant authority to commit the funds that will actually make the service available; if the HSA is to be responsible for the growth of services, it should also be responsible for reserving or allocating appropriate monies in support of the use of the services;
4. recognizes that whatever local authority is responsible for providing services should also be assured of payments for the approved services, not solely on the basis of use, but on the basis of availability; for example, the nursing home should not be dependent on full occupancy to generate maximum income; instead, if candidates for nursing home care can, in fact, be better served in a noninstitutional program, it should be made possible for the nursing home to keep beds in reserve, not be forced to solicit new patients or face economic distress because the long-term care continuum enables people to remain outside institutional care.

## Some Policy Issues

What is needed in long-term care today is a public policy that supports the individual's right to receive care, especially the right to expect that care is to be so coordinated and organized as to assure that it is appropriate. In the absence of such public policy, it is unrealistic to expect public support for a coordinated long-term care system. The Comprehensive Older Americans Act Amendments of 1978 do establish goals of comprehensive and coordinated service systems, but these are seen as expectations of federal agency cooperation rather than as a bill of rights for the older American. While they serve to notify organizational bureaucrats of their responsibility to cooperate in planning for the chronically ill, they do not clearly direct national policy.

Second, there is need for guaranteed funding to support the continuity of services in long-term care. The current method of funding does not designate the funds as dedicated to the recipient of services, which would implicitly support the premise that every person has a right to care. Rather, each service provider must assert its status and eligibility for payment before it can become part of the continuum. For example, adult day health services, an important service in the continuum, must develop a local funding plan wherever they operate in order to survive. Payments for existing programs usually come from a combination of Medicaid and Title XX of the Social Security Act. Older people cannot expect any adult day health service to be made available and paid for as an individual entitlement, but can receive services when providers and funding agencies acknowledge their eligibility to receive care. This is not entitlement.

Even if a basic core of services could be outlined to represent the minimum criteria of a continuum of long-term care, a continuum would not, in fact, exist unless it guaranteed that all the services would be available and a funded payment mechanism to purchase the service was in place. While the Comprehensive Older Americans Act Amendments of 1978 go further than any other public document to support the delivery of long-term care to all older Americans who need such services, the act itself does not establish services, provide for their funding on a regular basis, or require coordination of existing services. Either public policy must make a firmer statement of support for care programs, or services must somehow be implemented in the absence of supportive public policy. The latter alternative, implementing services to establish precedents, seems to be the only viable option in today's society. The continuum of long-term care under these circumstances will be whatever network of services the local community can generate within its existing resources. Obviously, in this system more affluent communities have the option of doing more. Conversely, rural and minority communities, often lacking adequate community resources, will be unable to establish a continuum of long-term care services.

To respond appropriately to the needs of frail older people, the service provider first must define and adopt concepts, philosophies, systems, and programs. The comprehensive system of long-term care services currently evolving has roots in a historical background of multiple, uncoordinated modes of care and multiple professional disciplines, but usually has been led by a single discipline. All of this is quite different from the contemporary notion of a "multidisciplinary" approach. Traditionally, long-term care has had diverse sponsorship and has been funded, generally inadequately, from a variety of uncoordinated sources, but could not be described as a cooperative venture.

In addition, it should be appreciated that the long-term care continuum, although defined as different from acute care, cannot be adequately conceptualized nor realistically implemented without understanding its relationship to the acute care system. Ultimately, it will be best for the patient and the continuity of patient care to have one single coordinated system of health and social services that includes acute and chronic care. Until that is achieved, we advocate integrating and clearly defining the parameters of an effective long-term care system with linkages to the acute care network.

Finally, the fact that some aspects of long-term care typically have been identified with poor quality has ramifications for issues of public expenditures for long-term care, assignment of responsibilities for establishing relevant standards for care and assuring their implementation, and appropriate preparation and training of employees in long-term care. A closely related issue is that of the ethical standards and commitment of everyone involved in the provision of long-term care.

Unquestionably, poor service in any aspect of long-term care should not be tolerated, but quality is not an inevitable by-product of lofty goals and good intentions. It must be maintained by responsible surveillance of the services, adequate measurable standards of performance, and enough resources to provide the expected services.

If long-term care as a total system is to advance from its current status of model or demonstration programs, the intent and content of the programs must be accepted into the mainstream of funding and administration policies of our health and social care systems. Obviously, major changes must occur at legislative and administrative levels.

Long-term care public policy should incorporate the following tenets:

First, there is a need for a national public policy supporting the contention that health care is a right of all persons, of all ages, of all ethnic backgrounds, and from all economic strata. While this policy may not immediately result in an equitable distribution of services for older people, it will set the stage for the incremental inclusion of services into the network of the continuum of care. Such public policy would also lend impetus to common efforts on behalf of the chronically ill by various federal agencies, thereby communicating a sense of self-worth to those who are chronically ill.

Second, it also is urgent that the spiral of chronic illness, with all of its complications, be reversed by dedicating appropriate resources of personnel, institutions, and finances to research into the causes and onset of chronic illness. The primary goal is to prevent or cure before disabilities are well entrenched. Programs in rehabilitation, especially those developed in the past twenty-five years, demonstrate that resources devoted to intensive rehabilitation immediately following an incident can result in greater productivity and greater life satisfaction. The person who benefits from early therapeutic intervention will be less dependent upon public support over long periods of time, and will therefore be less costly to society.

Third, it is important to recognize that long-term care, because it deals with individuals who have to accommodate their life styles to a chronic health problem, requires community responses that incorporate an understanding of both the nature of the health problems and the social ramifications of the chronic conditions. The care will be more effective if its providers understand and are sensitive to this total approach to human needs rather than supporting compartmentalization in which social care is vying with health care and specialists are trained to restrict their activities to one or the other of these fields. Such a separation invariably results in a schism in the care program, with the two care-giving groups ultimately vying for authority and control. The integrity of the individual is best supported by professionals who understand the importance of a holistic approach and support the resources necessary to maintain it. Such an approach to care can be initiated through multidisciplinary educational and work experiences.

Long-term care programs are currently offered under many auspices, with differing program goals and funding resources. In order to develop a comprehensive philosophy leading to a public policy in long-term care, it is essential to begin with a comprehensive statement of goals common to all service units comprising the continuum of care.

A statement of goals serves as the rallying point for everyone identified with the program, sets the stage for all participants to understand how their contributions can help achieve the goal, and serves as the base from which the program can be evaluated.

The goal statement prepared by the Federal Council on Aging (1978) is appropriate for long-term care programs for the frail elderly, and is offered as a guideline for public policy in long-term care. The goals of such care should be:

1. to assist the frail elderly to pursue reasonably independent and satisfying lives in their own places of residence;

2. to support frail elderly with apparent impairments, striving for a normalization of family and social relations by enabling such elderly to continue in their preferred environment, making critical decisions affecting their personal welfare;
3. to stimulate improved integration of preventive, ameliorative, and supportive health and social services from community-based, state, and national programs and resources;
4. to stabilize or eliminate actual or potential social isolation of the frail elderly without family or kin;
5. to utilize and integrate the respective contributions of family members and the formal helping network, along with efforts of the elderly for self help, to deal with the multiple needs of extended care associated with frailty in the later years;
6. to make more appropriate use of institutionalization so that such care will be reserved for those who clearly need it.

## Summary

The demographic changes in our population project increasing numbers of persons in the old old category, or those for whom there is the greatest probability of long-term chronic illness. In developing programs to meet the needs of those who are chronically ill, the first line of defense appears to be family and community support systems. Increasing efforts must be directed to strengthening these support systems to assure that those who are chronically ill have access to the personal, close caring of their families.

Long-term care as it is addressed here means more than institutional care or an unrelated segment of noninstitutional care. It refers to a coordinated network of services as well as the processes necessary to assess the particular needs of those who require such care and assure the appropriate use of the services. Long-term care is a forward looking approach to serving the increasing number of older people who are and will be in need of community services. The issues of appropriateness, coordination, assessment, and case management are all important to understanding the full potential of long-term care. Educational and preventive activities are directed to the maintenance of good health as well as the use of appropriate services when needed.

The ultimate effectiveness of long-term care depends on public policy that will communicate entitlements to those who are chronically ill. Each person should have the right to appropriate preventive and ameliorative services in the quality and quantity necessary to offset the disabling effects of chronic illness, if not the chronic illness itself.

Chapter

# 3

# The Components of Long-Term Care: A Historical Review

*A valuable lesson about long-term care can be gleaned from the experience of several European countries. Observations both of differences in approach from those used in the United States and of some similarities in problems provide a perspective on the issues that face us in this country.*

ROBERT L. KANE
ROSALIE A. KANE

## Attitudes Toward Aging

"History is not about the past alone. It is about change, with past and present in a mutual perspective. It clarifies the temporal context within which all of us must live, and helps us to understand the conditions of our existence" (Fischer 1979).

It is valuable to look back into the history of long-term care to evaluate the services that have been brought together as a continuum in which it is important to understand different backdrops, the history of each service, and the directions indicated for the future. It is especially important to understand history as we continue to seek ways to meld discrete services into a coordinated system without misunderstanding or misrepresenting each of the component parts, including institutional care, home health service, day care, service centers, and nutritional programs.

An examination of the history of aging would require an excursion too far back into the history of civilization to be appropriate here. Three useful books on the topic are *Aging, Its History and Literature,* by Joseph T. Freeman (1979); *Growing Old in America,* by David H. Fischer (1978); and *Old Age in the New Land,* by W. Andrew Achenbaum (1978).

The subject of aging is of great interest because it lies at the intersection of many major questions in our society about the family, the life cycle, morality, health care, public policy, welfare, taxes, and other issues. Because each of us is personally involved in an individual aging process, each of us has a stake in all the related societal issues that affect not only ourselves, but our parents, friends, children, and neighbors.

"Awareness of the nature of old age and the needs of the aging have a long lineage. The modern era began in 1909, when Ignatius Leo Hascher of New York coined the word 'geriatrics' for the clinical aspects of aging. Six years before that time, in 1903, I. I. Metchnikoff at the Pasteur Institute in Paris invented the term gerontology for the biological study of senescence" (Freeman 1979). Metchnikoff later won the Nobel Prize for his contributions to biology and the study of aging.

In the eighteenth century, Benjamin Rush discussed the clinical diseases of old age in a book in which he stressed heredity, temperance, mental vigor, equanimity, and marriage as pivotal factors in longevity. It was his early observation that few people die of old age; usually death in old age is the result of diseases (Freeman 1979). The search for answers to questions related to old age, the diseases of the aged, and the causes of deterioration and death continues today. "The drive toward extending the lifespan is as old as man. In its ultimate essence, the dream of the Fountain of Youth and eternal life is probably at the root of much religious belief. It is certainly behind the idea of rebirth and an eternal life beyond the grave. This drive never lets up and is probably based on a quality of the life phenomena, which is self-duplicating, persistent and, once started, apparently eternal" (Leeds 1964).

More recent additional efforts in the field of aging have been directed to the modification of social resources that relate to the quality of life for the older person. In preindustrial societies roles and status were frequently associated with the individual's age. "Industrial societies have tended to emphasize factors other than age for the assignment of roles, particularly in the adult years" (Friedman 1960). Today, old age is associated with a loss of status.

In addition to the changing roles of older persons and, "as a consequence of medical, technological and economic advances, a decline in mortality occurred, so that for the first time sizable numbers of people were living into their sixth decade or beyond" (Hendricks and Hendricks 1981). Prior to the end of the nineteenth century, while the social consciousness of several European governments had been awakened to the needs of the aged, "older people had a long time to wait before becoming a truly visible component of the American scene" (Hendricks and Hendricks 1981).

Friedman provided an example of the impact of early social thinking regarding care for the aging on the development of policy in the United States with the following:

> The Elizabethan Poor Law of 1601 represented a statement of public obligation for the support of the aged and disabled indigent through the establishment of public almshouses or through relief furnished to them in their own homes. It was to become the model for the New England poor laws and eventually set the pattern for most of our states. It was characterized by the almshouse, with its collection of petty thieves and unfortunates of all sorts, and the boarding-out system, in which the aged were auctioned off to the family who made the lowest bid for their care. The care of the indigent aged was early recognized as a community responsibility, but the manner in which the care was given defined their indigency as a mark of personal failure and unworthiness. (Friedman 1960)

Little community concern for the elderly was demonstrated in this country before the 1920s, when the disproportionate share of poverty among the aged was noted and pressures for social reforms were "directed toward the replacement of the traditional poorhouse with institutions more compatible with the needs of specific categories of dependents and, in the case of the aged, with the provision of pensions by the state or by industry" (Friedman 1960).

The 1920s also saw the assumption of philanthropic responsibilities by the middle class, with the development of women's groups, fraternal societies, and businessmen's clubs. These efforts led to the establishment of homes for the aged by the Moose Lodge, the Benevolent and Protective Order of Elks, the Independent Order of Odd Fellows, and labor unions and church groups (Friedman 1960).

In 1927 Abraham Epstein organized the American Association of Old Age Assistance to promote the notion of society's responsibility for the aged. This group became the American Association for Social Security in 1933. While the federal government had begun to assume a protective role over the rights of children in the early 1920s, it was not yet ready to respond to the needs of older persons. "What finally propelled the federal government into action on behalf of the elderly was in large part the result of the depression of the 1930s. For the first time in history, the American dream of an ever brighter tomorrow was challenged by the stark realities of economic blight" (Hendricks and Hendricks 1981).

The dramatic consequences of the economic depression required an examination of the issues of economic security related to age, disability, and retirement. Society's responsibilities shifted from providing temporary assistance in crisis situations to establishing a broader, more permanent framework of services designed to help individuals and groups attain reasonable standards of life and health (Friedman 1960). This was reflected in the establishment of social security and subsequent ongoing programs to sustain older people in society.

> The depression of the 1930s changed public welfare more than any other single episode in our history. In 1933, twenty-five million people in seven million households depended upon relief for their daily sustenance. The great depression saw the development of loan programs to the states for relief, rent programs, surplus commodity programs, public works programs, job training programs, and ultimately, the programs of the Social Security Act.
>
> The Social Security Act did two things: first, it established a natural retirement income system to provide income in lieu of wages to the worker or his dependents when the worker retired and (eventually) when he became disabled; second, it established a system of federal grants to states to provide financial assistance to the aged, dependent children, the blind, and the disabled. (Cohen 1974)

Additionally, the Social Security System gave older people the option to select and pay for the residence or care facility of their choice. While the amount of social security support was low, it did provide a minimum base of support, thereby reducing the need for public care of the elderly indigent and emphasizing care for those who were ill. Social Security gave the elderly some funds they could control, some measure of independence, and the ability to select services of their own choice. It is this same essential element of choice that underlies the development of long-term care into a continuum of services.

In the mid-1940s the commercial development of penicillin and other antibiotics, because of their effectiveness in treating infectious bacterial diseases, actually increased the chances that an elderly person would have to face chronic illness. Pneumonia, which had been known as the "friend of the aged" because the illness was almost always fatal, of short duration, and without handicapping complications, could now be cured. The new drugs enabled the elderly person to live longer and encounter some of the more disabling chronic illnesses instead of the quick death usually associated with acute illness.

Survival of the fittest has been displaced by survival of the chronically ill, thanks to antibiotics, and long-term care become a euphemism for care of the chronically ill. It would perhaps be more consistent to call contemporary long-term care centers by the names used to identify some of the earlier institutions, which did in fact refer to themselves as institutions for the incurable and chronically ill. Having been sensitized, however, to believing that, given the time, a cure can be found for all illnesses, we have come to view the term "incurable" as describing a condition that exists only for the time being. Those who are ill, care providers, and researchers all hope that scientific discovery will eventually remove the concept of "incurable" from our lexicon.

## Approaches to Treatment and Care

In 1951 an agency called Central Intake Service was officially opened by the Council on Care for the Aged and Chronic Sick of the Jewish Federation member agencies of Chicago. "Its purpose was to serve as the central point and the single agency within the system of Federation affiliates to which could come Jewish aged and/or their families desirous of help in the solution or alleviation of the personal and family problems which beset people in later life" (Katzen 1964).

This program recognized that "applications for home (institutional) admission represented a seeking for solutions to growing feelings of insecurity, fear of isolation and illness, need for protection, interfamilial difficulties, inadequate public agency services, and a variety of other problems. It was recognized that not all older people needed or wanted to live in institutions, that there were not sufficient numbers of beds available currently or in the foreseeable future to meet the demand" (Katzen 1964). Central Intake Service discovered that unless social service workers had the opportunity to understand and evaluate available resources in the community, the institutional setting was likely to be seen by them as the most effective way of dealing with a wide range of the problems of the elderly. "Central intake" has come to be known as "single point of entry" in long-term care. After almost thirty years of progress in the delivery of long-term care, one of the issues that still perplexes the most imaginative planners is developing a system of care that will encourage placement in an institution only when institutionalization is clearly preferable to noninstitutional services.

In 1977 the National Conference on Social Welfare, in its document *The Future For Long-Term Health Care in the United States,* identified as one of its dilemmas: "How to establish an intermediary system to perform specific tasks to expedite services more equitably and provide a continuum of care?" Its concern was to establish a case management system that would introduce the person into the appropriate service. The report argues that a comprehensive plan for complex health and social services needs to be developed, with control of entry into the system as an important tool for assuring appropriate care and control of cost.

Later in that year the New York State Communities Aid Association conducted an institute on long-term care. One of its recommendations dealt with the need to assist the chronically ill person with the choice of living and care arrangements, which was to be achieved by developing a network of services linked together by "gateway points of entry" (State Communities Aid Association 1977).

Callahan (1979) summarized the advantages of a single community-based agency for long-term care, and held out hope that "the existing problems of lack of access, inadequate resources, fragmentation, and high cost will be resolved somehow if only some way can be found to incorporate all aspects of long-term care into one agency."

A central issue in the development of such an agency is who controls entry into the system. For at least twenty-eight years—from 1951 to 1979—the literature reflects concern over this issue; of control of entry into the long term care system versus the maintenance of independent autonomous provider agencies. It is understandable that the issue has not yet been resolved, because it touches on the multiple forces of governments, issues in chronic illness, responsibility for the care of the chronically ill, funding, private agency jurisdiction, and some conceptual issues of autonomy, cooperation, and organization, as well as individual choice and privacy. It remains, however, as one of the most telling issues in the evolving long-term care continuum, an issue that must be resolved before an effective continuum can be established.

Newly introduced federally sponsored demonstration programs are intended to study further the effectiveness of the single point of entry into long-term care. These include the long-term care demonstration projects, channeling grants to states to improve the coordination of long-term care services, and the long-term care gerontology centers, university-based centers for research, education, and model developments.

## Institutional Care

In Europe, institutional programs to care for ill, handicapped, and needy persons were mainly the outgrowth of large charitable foundations and hospices, common from the twelfth to the eighteenth century (Dieck 1980): "The inhabitants of the charitable foundations received shelter, meals, and some of them nursing care; that is, the same services that still today, albeit in altered form, are offered in the institutions for the aged." In Germany, during the fifteenth and sixteenth centuries, there was a shift from care in institutions to care in the local community. A system of financial assistance was devised to deinstitutionalize the poorhouses, enabling the institutional residents to seek housing of their own choosing. In the nineteenth century, "the first homes devoted to caring for and nursing the elderly were established. The disability and old-age insurance law of 1889 allowed unattached, chronically ill, frail people seventy years of age and older the right to a place in a home if they relinquished their old-age pensions, and gave further impetus to this development (Dieck, 1980).

Early nursing homes in the United States derived from the European tradition of the almshouse or public poor house: Formalized health care in an institutional setting was initiated in this country in 1751, when the first hospital, The Pennsylvania Hospital, was founded. "It was followed soon thereafter by Philadelphia General, New York Hospital, and Bellevue. Each of these facilities had a poorhouse or almshouse as its progenitor. It wasn't until the latter part of the nineteenth century that any thought was given to reforming institutions for the sick and aged" (Moss and Halamandaris 1977). According to Cohen (1974), "While the last half of the nineteenth century was characterized by the fierce struggle for wealth and power, by the upheavals wrought by industrial development, urbanization, large scale immigration, widespread unemployment, and new economies, the almshouse continued in its central role in dealing with society's castoffs."

It was not until this century that private foundations, philanthropy, church support, and new immigrant aid societies gave rise to private voluntary organizations providing institutional care for the aged:

> The first Catholic home in the United States was the Lafon Asylum of the Holy Family established in 1842 in New Orleans, operated by the Sisters of the Holy Family, a negro congregation. Another religious order, the Sisters of the Third Order of St. Francis, began caring for sick elderly in their own homes at about the same time in Buffalo, New York, and in 1855 they established the St. Francis Home in Buffalo.
>
> Religious groups and national immigrant associations also were involved in establishing homes for aged in those years. The Home for Aged and Infirmed Israelites, the first known Jewish institution was founded in St. Louis in 1855 and almost

every national group of European origin, and even particular sections of various countries, established homes for aged, many of which continue at their old stands today.

A most prominent religious group involved with homes for aged is the Little Sisters of the Poor. This organization's first home in the United States was founded in Brooklyn in 1868. Later the same year other branches established homes in Cincinnati and New Orleans, and by 1874 there were thirteen homes under their auspices. (Gold and Kaufman 1970)

While homes for the aged were originally established for the poor, the changing perspective of poor laws, the advent of social security, and the impact of the introduction of antibiotic drugs led to the enlargement of the initial perspective to include people with chronic illness as well as those who had enough financial resources to choose a program and pay for the services provided.

Gold and Kaufman (1970), in their review of the history of homes for the aged, admonished readers that there was no need for the institutional environment to become a permanent-stay facility: "Deinstitutionalization of residents and repersonalization of patients have to be viewed as prime objectives on the road to humanizing the elderly people who stand in need of assistance, support, protection." From a more recent perspective, we should add that it is also important to avoid inappropriate institutionalization at the outset by providing care services essential to maintaining the individual at home. It is important to note that home care was probably available in this country a hundred years before there were institutional care programs. Despite that earlier beginning, however, home care still lags behind institutional care in the support it receives through public funds.

Institutional care has grown phenomenally since the 1930s. A 1939 Bureau of the Census report estimated there were 1,200 long-term care facilities in the United States, with 25,000 beds. A 1954 survey reported a total of 450,000 beds in 2500 homes. The rapid growth of institutional programs after World War II was stimulated further by the Medicare law of 1965, and resulted in an inventory of about 20,000 homes with a total capacity of almost one and a half million beds in the late 1970s (*Vital and Health Statistics* 1978). Projected growth for the year 2000 calls for close to two million beds.

## Rehabilitation

An important part of long-term care is the commitment to finding cures. "Cures" for chronic illnesses may include better ways of caring for those who are chronically ill, prevention of illnesses, and reversing or arresting their disabling impacts—for example, restoration of function following a stroke.

Since people are living longer today, they are more likely to develop chronic illnesses and concomitant disabilities. This trend has increased the importance of rehabilitation activities, which can restore physical and mental functions. "Rehabilitation" as a medical term dates back to 1918, but the concept is as old as Hippocrates' prescription of leather shoes for children born with a clubfoot. His aphorism, "Exercise strengthens and inactivity wastes" is a basic principle of rehabilitation.

According to Moss (1974), "the first objective of rehabilitation medicine is to eliminate the physical disability if that is possible; the second, to reduce or alleviate the disability to the greatest extent possible; and the third, to retrain the person with a residual physical disability to live and work within the limits of the disability, but at the maximum of his capabilities" (Moss 1974).

In the 1940s, physicians acknowledged the medical significance of early ambulation, thereby offsetting many of the complications of prolonged bed rest. Following World War II the treatment of physically disabled persons improved markedly (Riffle 1973). At the war's end, rehabilitation was an accepted part of military and Veterans Administration hospital care, but remained very limited for the nonmilitary. In 1948 a rehabilitation center was established at New York University College of Medicine which later (1951) became the Institute of Physical Medicine and Rehabilitation (Moss 1974).

The concepts of rehabilitation, and especially the professions of physical therapy and occupational therapy, found their ways into the long-term care field in the later 1950s and early 1960s. Their principles helped shift emphasis from the passive notions of a "rest home" or rest as a treatment for disabilities to active rehabilitation programs in long-term care institutions. This was followed by rehabilitation approaches to restoring mental functioning and the development of programs such as reality orientation and remotivation, which became standard services in long-term care institutions.

## Home Health Services

The advent of home health care can be traced back to the Boston Dispensary, which in 1796 gave those who were sick and poor the dignity of being cared for in their homes rather than in the hospital. In 1877 the Woman's Branch of the New York City Mission was the first establishment in the United States to hire a graduate nurse to provide nursing care for the sick in their homes. In 1885 the first voluntary agency (nongovernment) specifically organized to provide home nursing care was founded in Buffalo, New York. Other voluntary agencies, later to become Visiting Nurse Associations, opened their doors in Boston and Philadelphia in 1886 (Stewart 1979). While the early home care programs were run by volunteers, in 1898 the Los Angeles County Health Department became the first official health department to hire graduate nurses.

Visiting nurse services became the primary provider of home health services in the northeastern United States, with the public health agencies assuming responsibility in the west and south. In more recent years, disciplines other than nursing have added to the panoply of in-home services, including social services, physical therapy, nutrition, speech and occupational therapy, and home-maker-home health aides. These evolved into what is now called a comprehensive coordinated home care program. Home health care became more pervasive when, "In the late 1940s, hospitals began to enter the home health care field. This interest in home care occurred after the discovery of antibiotics and implementation of immunization programs. These two factors were largely responsible for the shift in health care programs from acute communicable disease to chronic illness, a change also reflected in the health care delivery system" (Stewart 1979).

One of the best known hospital-based home care programs was the Montefiore Hospital Home Care Program developed in New York City in 1947, which included a wide range of medically and socially oriented home care services (Cherkosky 1949).

The Medicare and Medicaid programs initiated in 1965 provided for reimbursement of selected health care services given in the home and set specific guidelines that home health agencies had to meet in order to be eligible for reimbursement. Of great importance was the "nursing plus one" requirement that home health agencies provide at least one other specified service in addition to nursing.

However, Trager (1972) finds severe limitation in home health services in the United States and in the policies of Medicare and Medicaid.

> The availability of comprehensive home health services in the United States could substantially affect the appropriate utilization of all health care resources. Such comprehensive services are not available at the present time. The potential broad community-based home health programs capable of serving large population groups with varying and fluctuating needs has barely been demonstrated. Hospital-based programs are also in short supply and are not being developed in proportion to need. Focused upon short-term concentrated care, they do not have available for the community those services which can be extended to meet long-range need. Home health services, where they do exist, are underfinanced, limited in their capacity to

cover the population in need, frequently lacking in essential components which might make them an effective resource.
>They are diminishing in numbers.
>They are curtailing their services.
>They are narrowing their coverage to selected population groups.
>They are reducing the duration of the care they offer.

Trager continues her critique with comments about home health aides: "Homemaker-home health aide programs which should supply the essential basic supports when family members are not capable of supplementing care—or when there are no family members—are rare. They are limited in their ability to meet population demand either for short- or long-term care."

With regard to the issue of accessibility of home health services, Trager says, "There are geographic areas of the country and large sections of the population which do not have home health services of any kind available. Services are fragmented, geared to special groups, underfinanced, diminished as the need increases."

Discussing the quality of home health services, Trager says, "The auspices under which the services are provided do not determine their quality. Whether hospital-based, community-based, or existing in an assembly of community agencies, each offering the components of home health care has essential features which are described as 'good quality' and offer *all* of the needed services that must be available to all the population. Such services must be available in a supply which is adequate for the population. They must be coordinated, whether they are under a single roof or housed and administered separately. They must provide a network which continuously provides services for as long as they are needed."

Home health services and home health agencies are not considered synonymous terms. The first is a concept based upon clearly defined standards of excellence, as any health care institution of good quality must be. The second is a legislative title which includes only selected and expedient elements of home health services.

In January 1975 there were approximately 2,247 (National League for Nursing 1975) certified home health agencies in the United States. The majority were voluntary or public agencies which had offered home care services prior to passage of the Medicare insurance legislation, i.e., they were not substantially new resources responding to the increased need for home health services. Generally, home health services for the older person have been limited by the short supply of programs and do not provide more than the "nursing plus one" services. They fail to respond adequately to the myriad needs of older persons and are mired down in the paper requirements of the Medicare program. These failings inhibit home health services from becoming the mainstay of long-term care and the primary resource enabling older people to remain at home.

In 1977 the comptroller general of the United States submitted a report to the Congress titled "Home Health—The Need for a National Policy to Better Provide for the Elderly." The report found that "home health care and related home services for the elderly are not effectively coordinated," and that what is required is an overall federal policy for home health care. Only in the presence of such a policy could programs be consolidated and more effectively coordinated to serve the needs of the elderly population.

Under current laws, home health care is supported primarily under Medicare, Medicaid, Title XX, and the Older Americans Act. Differing eligibility requirements, services, and responsibilities for research, demonstrations, and evaluation create a sense of underlying confusion in the administration of home care programs. Additionally, some home care programs are sponsored by public health departments or receive community support through the United Way or other fund raising efforts. The comptroller's report concluded that: "Services are available through so many different programs that effective coordination and delivery of home health and other in-home services seems close to impossible." It also added that, "Services provided are not accessible through a single entry point. Interagency/intra-agency agreements between federal, state and local agencies have not provided effective coordinated services to beneficiaries." Further, the report recommended "that the Secretary of HEW develop a national policy to be considered by the Congress which would consolidate home health activities. HEW should promote the establishment of a comprehensive single entry system by which the needs of patients are assessed prior to their placement in a program."

In Michigan, at the Saginaw Hospital, home care is combined with day care. Essentially bed-bound patients are brought to the hospital's rehabilitation department by special bus. There they receive social services, rehabilitative, and dental services in a day care setting. At the same time or subsequent to the day care, patients are provided skilled nursing and home health aide services in their own homes. This admixture of day care and home care can be modified as the patient improves, decreasing the amount of time spent in the day care center and increasing the time spent at home until the patient reaches his maximum level of independence. (Ryder, Stitt, and Elkin 1969)

## Adult Day Health Services

In the early history of day health services, distinctions were made between the day hospital and day care center. The first day hospitals were developed for psychiatric patients, and the model of day hospitals for elderly patients with physical disabilities and illnesses was established at the Crowley Road Hospital, Oxford, England, in 1958 (Lorenze, Hamill, and Oliver 1974). "A day hospital is a model for providing health and supportive services to patients. It is operated by or is part of a general or special hospital. Patients who come to the program, one or more times per week, spend a major portion of the day at the day hospital and return home to spend the night" (Lorenze, Hammill, and Oliver 1974).

Day care services are defined as:

> Services whereby patients are transported, often in specially equipped vehicles, to a common setting for purposes of receiving medical-nursing and health-related social services with the aim of helping them attain physical rehabilitation or maintain their current physical status. Patients may spend from several hours to a full eight or more hours in the day care facility for a period of one to five days a week. Day care may be provided under the auspices of a hospital, nursing home or extended care facility. The services of the day care facility are often merged with the operation of the sponsoring facility and usually include physical therapy, occupational therapy, speech therapy, group therapy, specific nursing procedures, dentistry, podiatry, and personal care. The aim of day care services is to dissociate the "hotel" element of hospital care from therapeutic content, leaving only the latter. (U.S. D.H.E.W. 1972)

The similarity between the definitions of day hospital and day care suggests that there is a range of social and medical care services that can be provided in either setting without regard to the title. In fact, more recently the title "adult day health services" has been recommended for the services offered under the rubric of either day care or day hospital (Trager 1979). Services provided in adult day health services vary along a continuum from active rehabilitation to solely physical and social maintenance with services assisting the client in the activities of daily living.

Some of the earlier day care programs in this country were organized in terms of several different approaches: networks of centers, centers associated with other health care facilities, freestanding programs related to other health networks, and freestanding independent programs. The earliest known program still functioning is the Adult Day Treatment Center established under private auspices in 1965 in Beverly Hills, California (Directory of Adult Day Care Centers 1978).

In 1967 a network of day care centers located in four hospitals and two nursing homes was established by the Handmaker Jewish Nursing Home for the Aged in Tucson, Arizona, and was the nation's largest system of geriatric day care services (Lamden and Greenstein 1975). In the same year the Mansfield Home in Mansfield, Ohio, initiated its day care program; and in 1969 St. Otto's Nursing Home Day Care Program was established in Minnesota. The Levindale Day Care Program was opened and became the first "subacute care" facility in New York State to be licensed for outpatient services (Melita and Mach 1975).

The On Lok Senior Day Health Center, opened in San Francisco in 1973, was "established as one link in a planned chain of services and programs needed to maintain the frail elderly in the community at a maximum level of functioning. It serves three principal ethnic groups of residents in the city's Chinatown–North Beach area—Chinese, Filipino, and Italian-American—as well as other elderly. The focus is on health care, physical and occupational therapy for rehabilitation and maintenance, social services and nutrition, with therapies delivered by a bilingual professional and paraprofessional staff seven days a week" (Lurie et al. 1976).

Fewer than fifteen day care programs existed in the entire nation before 1973; today it is estimated that there are nearly six hundred such programs, of varying content and emphasis (Trager 1979). It is difficult to determine how many of these programs approximate the definition of services described by Trager. The absence of consistent licensing or certifying criteria, and especially the difficulty in obtaining consistent funding for day care, hinders the development of high standards and expansion of the number of this important service.

In the fall of 1977, California became the first state to pass legislation mandating payment for adult day care through Title XIX of the Social Security Act. Typically, programs are funded through Titles XVIII, XIV, and XX of the Social Security Act, the Older Americans Act, revenue sharing, United Way, and direct payments by participants. In 1978 Title XX was used to fund 135 programs in thirty-five states, and Title XIX funded 47 programs in four states while also providing partial funding of some aspects of the program such as physical therapy (Directory of Adult Day Care Centers 1978).

In 1977, with support from the National Center for Health Services Research, the University of Arizona sponsored two workshops attempting to clarify the status of adult day health services. Participants concluded, among other things, that:

> The principle that adult day health care is not a single service but a range of services provided in a variety of settings that represent part of the community care continuum, inextricably bound into the community support system—and that adult day health care is a modality which offers an as-yet-unrealized

(on a national scale), but invaluable, new resource to vulnerable populations for whom there is at present no care resource or none as potentially effective. (Trager 1979)

One of the new resources provided by adult day health programs is the social setting in which functional assessments can be made of the older person's daily living activities and social skills. This latest effort in adult health services clearly is a vital component in the long-term care continuum.

## Senior Centers

In contrast to the core of health care services essential to the adult day health services, the senior center builds upon the social functioning of its participants to develop a variety of social, recreational, educational, civic, and health related activities. Many people who grow old in the United States become isolated, removed from relatives and friends. "The Senior Center of today is a community focal point on aging, a place where older persons can meet together, receive services, and participate in activities that will enhance their dignity, support their independence, and encourage their involvement in and with the community" (Leanse, Tiven, and Robb 1977). The senior center has been an important link in the continuum of long-term care because it can assume responsibility for many of the educational, preventive, and advocacy issues on behalf of the elderly. These activities, while not necessarily serving the frail elderly, are an important part of the continuum that attempts to maintain the independent functioning of older people and, through its services, reduce the disabilities of loneliness and isolation.

The first senior center in New York City, the William Hodson Community Center, was established in 1943. This was followed by the San Francisco Senior Center in 1947, Little House in Menlo Park, California, in 1949, and the Philadelphia Center for Older People in 1954. A recent directory of senior centers (1974) lists nearly five thousand clubs and senior centers in the United States. According to one report, these are centers which,

although starting from different perspectives and serving different clienteles, have as their basic goal to provide the means to develop the potential inherent in older people.

The growth of Centers, however, closely corresponds to the flow of federal dollars made available to Senior Centers after passage of the 1965 Older Americans Act. Other federal agencies began to channel dollars into older person programs, enabling many senior centers to expand programs directed to the elderly of minority groups previously unserved or underserved by largely activity-focused programs. The federally sponsored nutrition program has increased the number of sites for older person services and activities. (Leanse, Tiven, and Robb 1977)

The 1973 and 1978 Amendments to the Older Americans Act of 1965 provide for training for center personnel, technical assistance, and advocacy on behalf of centers.

The relationship of the senior center to adult day health programs is much like that between congregate housing and nursing homes. The senior center, when viewed as part of the continuum of long-term care, responds to the needs of the older person able to participate in a self-directing program. Participants in adult day health services are in need of specific health interventions that assist in rehabilitation or restorative activities. Residents of congregate housing live semi-independently because they can take advantage of the resources of the housing program, unlike the occupants of nursing homes, who reside in that environment because they are unable to live independently.

## Congregate Housing

Congregate housing provides an environment that encourages and supports older persons to be as independent as they are able. Under certain circumstances it enables them to remain outside of institutional environments which provide more intensive medical services.

Congregate housing is an age-segregated, integrated housing and service package in a noninstitutional environment. Public housing for the elderly preceded the development of congregate housing.

It was not until the Housing Act of 1956 that the basic legislation for public housing was modified to accommodate the specific problems of the elderly. The Housing Act of 1956 authorized the construction of new housing (or remodeling of existing housing) specifically designed for elderly families. In 1959 the first federal subsidized private housing program of any kind was enacted; it was specifically designated for the elderly. Section 202 of the Housing Act of 1959 introduced a private direct loan program for the purpose of providing housing for the elderly. (Welfeld 1978)

One of the first federal programs to produce housing designed especially for elderly or handicapped Americans was Section 202 of the Housing Act of 1959, intended to stimulate new multifamily housing construction. This program made loans available to nonprofit sponsors, and was designed to provide independent living for elderly and handicapped persons.

A substantial amount of new construction has been developed for the elderly under Section 8 of the Housing and Community Development Act of 1974, and also under a revised form of Section 202, called Section 202/8.

The Congregate Housing Services Act of 1978 promoted the coordination of supportive services, with congregate housing as the means of maintaining independence for those temporarily disabled or handicapped. The importance of integrating a wide range of social services for the elderly into the physical dwelling place is seen as one component of a mix of factors required to enable the elderly to achieve dignified independent living. In one survey, health-related services were most frequently requested by tenants of congregate housing, with meal services and housekeeping or chore services ranking close behind. (Gutowski 1978)

The needs of older people cannot be adequately met by housing alone; the housing must be accompanied by appropriate services. In some situations, housing for the elderly has been developed together with or in proximity to senior centers, nutrition programs, or other health-related services to make such services readily accessible.

## Nutrition Services

The final report of the White House Conference on Food, Nutrition and Health in 1970 left little doubt that a significant number of older people in the United States are malnourished. It is likely that from eight to ten million of those over sixty-five in 1970 suffered from malnutrition, with many of these older people living in social isolation in or near poverty: "Nutrition is more than food, and perhaps more acutely so with older persons as life term diminishes and characteristics of daily living increasingly relate to deprivation. Significant are: motivation toward eating, customary and cultural attitudes and practices, general mental and physical health, isolation, availability of food, geography, transportation, economics, and education in the use of food" (Weg 1978).

Weg also describes four ways that nutrition can affect aging. First, good nutrition is endangered by disabilities, loneliness, transportation barriers, and decreased income. Second, malnutrition abets the development of some diseases that accompany old age. Third, in ways that are not yet entirely known, nutrition may affect the nature and rate of aging. Fourth, nursing home attendants may, due to neglect, ignorance, or understaffing, fail to address the wide-ranging factors that relate to nutritional adequacy.

The issue of nutrition is raised here because the problems of poor or limited nutrition among older persons gave rise to a variety of nutritional programs that have, over time, become a very significant part of long-term care services.

Specialized meal programs began under voluntary auspices in the early 1950s, and consisted mostly of meals-on-wheels programs. "Senior centers and clubs often provided hot meals at a common site. Such programs, however, were but one component of other services. It was not until the 1973 Comprehensive Service Amendments to the Older Americans Act that federal policy provided funding for nutritional services for the aging. The emphasis was on the establishment of local sites for congregate dining services to provide nutritionally sound meals for older persons" (Beattie 1976). The Title VII Nutritional Program for the Elderly was part of the 1972 Amendments to the Older Americans Act and was intended to promote a "national policy which provides older Americans, particularly those with low incomes, with low cost, nutritionally sound meals served in strategically located centers such as schools, churches, community centers, senior citizens centers, and other public or private nonprofit institutions where they can obtain other social and rehabilitative services."

The socialization and nutrition programs funded under the Older Americans Act have been relatively successful programs because of the large numbers served (72, 167, 480 in 1981), as well as the prevention and outreach aspects of the total program. The nutrition sites often serve as the primary entry point into the long-term care system, especially for those not presenting medical care as the primary need. Additionally, the relationship between transportation to nutrition sites and the nutrition programs creates a daily opportunity for overseeing the clients' home situations and assuring that alternate home services are made available if the individual cannot come to the nutrition site. The content of programs provided through the nutrition sites can be part of a planned approach to preventive health care, and can encourage those served to be aware of their own needs, of their rights to have some of those needs met, and of the services available for doing so. The nutrition site and its related programs provide a valuable opportunity to assess the needs of the older person. The amendments of the Older Americans Act of 1978 coordinated existing Title VII nutrition programs with other Title III programs—namely, the area agency on aging and senior centers—putting the nutritional programs in the mainstream of community programs for the elderly.

## The Continuum of Long-Term Care

The Amendments to the Older Americans Act of 1971 introduced the concept of "area wide model projects" as demonstration programs designed to provide needed services to elderly persons living at home that would postpone or prevent their having to be admitted to a nursing home. Funds were provided to help communities design and test innovative ways of assisting the elderly continue their independent living as long as possible.

An early demonstration program was developed in Tucson (Pima County), Arizona, by the Pima Council on Aging in 1972. The program continued until 1976, when its services were taken over by Pima County Government as a permanent function of the county care system. Central to the delivery system was the concept that each person participating in the program would be assigned a facilitator—a social worker responsible for identifying what services were needed, arranging for service delivery, and monitoring appropriateness of care. The services selected as most critically needed by Pima County residents aged fifty-five or older or at risk of institutionalization were health-homemaker, home delivered meals, socialization and nutrition, day care, and transportation (McEvers 1976).

In 1975, the Monroe County (New York) long-term care program known as "Access" was developed with a demonstration grant entitled "A Demonstration of Community-wide Alternative Long Term Care Model." This program was funded under the Section 1115 Medicaid provisions to support programs that would help reduce increasing Medicaid costs. The program was designed to make long-term care services most appropriate, most cost effective, and most acceptable to the clients. Case management was included in the program, and was to be "an administrative service defined as the management of a process that includes the coordination of a comprehensive preadmission assessment. Also included was the development and approval for payment of a service plan, the initiation of home services or placement assistance, and the monitoring of a follow-up procedure" (*Monroe County Long-Term Care Program* 1979).

In 1973, the Chelsea-Village Program of St. Vincent's Hospital on the lower west side of Manhattan initiated a prototype hospital-based home health care program for homebound, isolated, aged people. Other programs, such as Triage, of Plainville, Connecticut; the Senior Care Action Network (SCAN) of Long Beach, California; and Texas Research Institute of Mental Health (TRIMS), were developed as the product of local community efforts to embrace several levels of care within a coordinated system of services for the elderly.

According to Beattie (1976): "The evolution of the long-term care continuum can assure continuity of care as well as the full range of services which are prevention, treatment, and rehabilitation oriented. . . . Such centers usually combine service functions, research functions, and training functions which enable them not merely to respond to the needs of the present day aging but also to build knowledge out of practice in order to modify old services and anticipate the need for new services."

The 1978 Amendments to the Older Americans Act of 1965 committed the Commissioner on Aging "to strengthen the involvement of the Administration in the development of policy alternatives in long-term care and to insure that the development of community alternatives is given priority attention"; further, "to encourage and assist state and local agencies to concentrate resources in order to develop greater capacity and foster the development of comprehensive and coordinated service systems to serve older individuals . . ." (US Department HEW, *Comprehensive Older Americans Act Amendments of 1978*). This act served as the stimulus for the development of long-term care gerontology centers where education, training, service, and research in long-term care will be coordinated to enhance the effectiveness of long-term care services.

## The Challenge to Long-Term Care

A historical review of long-term care illustrates that it was not until the 1950s that social policies, programs, and services to meet the specialized needs of the aging began to emerge. The momentum in this direction was heightened in the 1960s, when the landmark Medicare and Older Americans Act laws were passed, but gaps still exist between the size of the rapidly growing older segment of our society and the public policies and programs essential to keep pace with the needs of this group.

It is evident that multiple levels of services, with options and alternatives, are required to respond to the unique and changing needs of older people. Where few services exist, it is not possible to provide alternatives and choice (Beattie 1976). Multiple services in sufficient quantity and of acceptable quality require more public funds than have so far been allocated to meet these needs. Coordinated services, centralized intake, and case management all increase the need for funds and therefore require a change in public policy.

Another important issue is the role of the institution in the continuum of care. Institutions are currently seen by many as last resorts for the elderly, but this assumes that institutionally-based and community-based systems are mutually exclusive. In fact, there is an appropriate place for institutions in the continuum of services.

In addition, there is a need to determine whether the traditional health care system should be supplemented by creating social care systems that aim to keep the chronically ill older person functioning within the community. This calls for the development within the coordinated health care system of a wide range of housing services, home health services, and other social services that respond to the needs of the chronically ill through current services, preventive care, and research. Achievement of this goal will not preclude the need for institutional services of a high quality for the frail and infirm or acute care for those with acute episodes of illnesses (Kane and Kane 1976).

It seems important to repeat again that long-term care, if it is to be effective for any older person, should be available to everyone, and that a public policy assuring universal access to health care is the basic prerequisite for a rational delivery program.

In 1972 Steinfeld outlined five basic principles that should serve as the cornerstone of a national health care policy. These included:

1. Equal access to health care for all. Racial, ethnic, social, and geographic barriers must be eliminated or minimized.
2. Supply and demand must be reasonably balanced.
3. The health care system must be organized efficiently. Placing the burden of meeting the greater new demands generated by increased funding on the same old inefficient system is fatal.
4. The existing strengths of our system should be used as a foundation instead of being discarded.
5. Programs should be based on health—not health care alone. Individuals should be encouraged to act responsibly in their daily lives through programs of health education, health maintenance, and disease prevention.

This challenge could very well serve as the challenge to long-term care today for the issues of access to care, supply and demand, and organization of services are especially significant in long-term care policy. Programs of long-term care should not be based on health care alone, but rather should be based on health and on helping maintain those who are chronically ill in the best possible condition and circumstances.

## Policy Issues

According to Binstock and Levin (1976), "The fundamental notion that governments should intervene in the social condition of aging persons has been firmly established in industrialized societies. . . . Yet, accompanying the growing commitment of modern societies to public intervention for the solution of social problems is a deepening sense of despair over our seeming incapacity to intervene effectively." These authors continue to say that the "onus for our despair rests in part with theoretical and empirical inadequacies in our capacity to develop and design effective modes of social intervention." Clearly, long-term care must fit into the category of inadequately designed modes of social intervention despite historical references that give evidence of efforts of social intervention on behalf of the elderly and chronically ill. But, if as Lipman (1979) says, "The family is the primary support system of the elderly person," the family's own examination of social intervention strategies must also conclude that the absence of strategies that would enable them to assume the role of major support of the older person may have contributed to that "deepening sense of despair" and our inability to "intervene effectively."

A review of some of the major public policies related to older people, and especially to long-term care, will give evidence of the broad scope of public intentions. A complete list of these programs is included in the Appendix. Major public programs having an important impact on long-term care include: the Social Security Act of 1935, establishing the policies of retirement insurance and old age assistance; Titles XVIII, XIX, and XX Amendments to the Social Security Act, providing financial resources for health and social services; the Older Americans Act of 1965, and its subsequent amendments pronouncing the broad expectations of public policy and aging, and funding some measure of educational programs, research, and demonstrations; the National Health Planning and Resources Development Act of 1974, establishing the Health Systems Agencies and delineating their responsibilities for regulating the development of licensed health care services. The execution of public policy, emanating from different agencies, with different authorities and interests, and without any real central authority, has been one source of difficulty in evolving a clear program direction for long-term care. Funds, authority to regulate, and program development must be coordinated to meet the needs of the population of chronically ill older people.

# Summary

Butler (1978) has described how our own attitudes toward aging affect planning and implementation of long-term care:

> . . . beneath the historical changes in the roles and status of the aged is an underlying and apparently universal ambiguity in people's attitudes toward aging. Understandably, there is both fear and distaste for the decline of the "self" with time. This fear is not easily overcome, even in a new land of plenty . . . Attitudes toward the aged are once again in flux, and many sectors of our population have taken new interest in this large minority: new programs for older citizens, new centers for the elderly, apartment buildings specially designed to meet the needs of the aged—all of these are indications of the impact the elderly have on our society. What also seems clear, therefore, is that the situation can be improved: once society understands the genesis of its negative attitudes, it can begin to move toward meeting the needs of older people through legislative initiatives on income maintenance, health care, housing, and research.

While some forms of programs related to the elderly were attempted early in our history, communal responses to the needs of the chronically ill seem to have emerged after the mid-1940s, following the introduction of antibiotic medicines. Prior to that, institutional care was the primary method of attending to the poor, the homeless, and the chronically ill. Senior centers were introduced in 1943, the concept of central intake appeared in 1951, the first hospital-based home care program in 1954, specialized housing for the elderly in 1956, and adult day health care in 1965. The Medicare and Medicaid amendments to the Social Security Act and the Older Americans Act, both of 1965, gave considerable impetus to the development of and funding of programs for the chronically ill and there have been major increases in services during the past fifteen years.

Yet there is still no comprehensive national policy, no vehicle for coordinating the multiple governmental and non-governmental programs, and no organized community delivery system to assure that appropriate services are responsive to the needs of the chronically ill. The situation is improving. Most noteworthy are efforts to develop local, community-based, long-term care systems; support systems to encourage family involvement in care of the chronically ill; long-term care demonstration programs; and long-term care gerontology centers to be located on campuses throughout the country, coordinating research, education, and model developments.

# Chapter
# 4

# Defining
# the Components
# of
# Long-Term Care

*If we can design a system of long-term care based on the needs of the individual (through a unified system of entitlements) then the institution will take its rightful place as a specialized facility providing organized services unavailable elsewhere to the elderly at-risk population. If the long-term care facility did not exist we would have to invent it, but as it is we need to refine the system and cast it in a new mold.*

HERBERT H. SHORE

The older person in need of services is less likely to be interested in concepts, philosophy, systems, or definitions than in finding out how to get a needed service when it is required. If the appropriate services are not available, the person will want to know why. The complications of chronic illness make it difficult to present quick solutions to any problem, even when "solution" is broadly defined as any response beyond the expression of a desire to mitigate the disabilities of chronic illnesses.

Long-term care is not determined by the length of time over which services are provided, but rather by the extent of chronicity of the illness—the expectation that the intruding disability will not be eliminated by the health care intervention. It is expected that accommodation to the chronic health care condition will draw on personal resources, family support and other social contacts, the social environment, and the service system.

The frail elderly are defined by the Federal Council on Aging (1978) as the "oldest of older Americans with an accumulation of health, social, economic, and environmental problems which impede their independent living to the extent that they need continuing personal assistance." This group constitutes the majority of occupants of nursing homes, and is the group for whom "alternatives to institutional care" are sought. These people cannot on their own arrange for improved responses, adequate funding, and protection of individual rights. They are therefore dependent upon others for active support and community concern.

This group also includes large numbers of people who are living at home but are often ignored there. The social needs of the frail elderly are given too little attention in the present health care system. "Careful estimates from household surveys are that 12 percent to 14 percent of the population sixty-five years of age and over can be left by themselves for only short periods of time. . . . As would be expected with advancing age, the proportion of the 'very sick' increased from 9 percent for the age group sixty-five to seventy-four, to 14 percent among persons seventy-five years and over. . . ." (Anderson 1976). In order to understand the full scope of the problem, these numbers should be added to those for the institutionalized population, which is 5 percent of those over sixty-five and about 14 percent of those over seventy-five years of age.

## Some Statistics on the Frail Elderly

About two million to three million older people living at home have physical or mental limitations that require them to have help from family, friends, or social agencies to perform the ordinary tasks of daily living.

The most frequently reported chronic conditions and impairments for the elderly living outside of institutions (Brotman 1978) are: arthritis (38 percent); vision and hearing problems (20 percent); and heart conditions and hypertension (20 percent). The primary causes of death among the over sixty-five population are, by rank: heart disease (44 percent); cancer (19 percent); strokes (13 percent); and influenza and pneumonia (3 percent).

The sickest of the elderly generally reside in the nation's approximately 18,300 nursing homes. These elderly individuals, about 4 percent to 5 percent of the elderly population, suffer from multiple chronic conditions. Almost two-thirds are significantly mentally impaired, 36 percent have heart problems, and 14 percent suffer from diabetes. Almost a third are confined to beds or chairs.

Almost one-half cannot see well enough to read an ordinary newspaper even if they wear glasses. Thirty-five percent cannot hear a conversation on an ordinary telephone, and 24 percent have impaired speech (Iglehart 1978).

It is important to note that the presence of any of these impairments or of any group of impairments in combination is not sufficient evidence of the need for institutionalization, or even for a full range of supportive services at home. Individuals respond differently to the same problems and accommodate their lifestyles in very personal ways. The presence of physical, emotional, or social problems needs to be viewed from the perspective of the person beset with the problems, the accommodation made to the problems, and the supports available in the social and physical environments.

More than any other population group, the chronically ill elderly need and use medical care. They not only spend the most money on it, but they have the lowest incomes and the least adequate private health insurance coverage. Per capita annual personal health expenditures for those sixty-five and older was $1,745 in fiscal 1977, compared with $661 for those aged nineteen to sixty-four and $253 for persons under nineteen. In 1976, Medicare financed seventy-one percent of the hospitalization of its beneficiaries and fifty-five percent of their care by physicians. Altogether, public programs paid for 67 percent of the personal health care expenses of the elderly in fiscal 1977. Yet, it is important to note that during this same period, less than 3 percent of Medicare's expenditures was used to pay for home health care (Iglehart 1978).

Because, in the arena of public funding, institutional care has been favored over home care, home care and the related elements of a coordinated continuum of long-term care have not flourished. The following statement about services in the continuum proposes a theoretical framework for the organization of the full network of long-term care services into a coordinated program. Core services, or those services that are the essential foundation should be an entitlement of all persons who because of the presence of a disabling chronic illness require the appropriate assessment and case management—both core services—in order to gain access to the most appropriate care program. An obvious corollary of the concept of core services as entitlements is that public funds must be made available to support these services.

## Services in the Continuum

### Core Services

Services of an effective long-term care system that should be available to all candidates as entitlements include: information, referral, outreach, multidisciplinary assessment centers, and case management. The availability and use of the core services should enable the person in need to obtain the prescription for services that best responds to the total needs presented. It then is the case manager's job to assist the individual and family in obtaining the services and identifying potential sources for payments.

Individuals' needs will vary as they make application for long-term care services. Variations of need will depend upon the degree of impairment, dependency, and availability of supportive resources. The older person should be helped to remain at home with supports if this is his or her desire, and if that choice is feasible. The continuum has been defined earlier as the close union of related parts of a service system, including services offered at home, in nonresidential service centers, in housing programs, and in institutional facilities. This perspective differs from other conceptualizations of the continuum that describe only two options for service, the home or institution. The varying combinations of resources and four specific options for service arrangements are described below.

## The Integrated Home and Service Center Model

In this arrangement, the person can continue in his or her own household, with its familiarity, conveniences, security, and related neighbor social structure, if these resources are available. This alternative is effective for the person who is able to leave the household and travel to the service center but is, of course, dependent upon transportation resources. The service center is not viewed separately from the home, but rather as an integrated adjunct within the network. The service center assumes primary responsibility for the delivery of a variety of health and social services, as well as for noticing any changing functional capacities that may make it necessary to introduce additional home supports. For this alternative to be workable, the service centers must be nearby and convenient to residences. Service centers may be senior centers, nutrition sites, health centers, private practitioners' offices, or any other organization providing these services.

Family supports are welcomed in this arrangement, since the older person remains relatively independent and not constrained in movement or activity by the living arrangements. Additionally, the close interrelationship between the home and service center can serve as an aid to the family, both in providing care and in teaching the family to understand the changing functioning of the older person so the family can participate effectively in appropriate care. In reality, however, there is limited funding available for this level of service—a situation directly contradictory to the notion that money spent early in support, education, and preventive measures will probably be cost-effective if more intensive services or institutionalization can be postponed or avoided.

In this model, while the older person continues to live at home, either alone or with others, most of the services are delivered outside the home. The service package can vary, and the older person is urged to assume primary responsibility for his or her own care as well as for the services from family or the service center.

This model is dependent upon a close relationship between a service agency and the individual in need of services, and offers the greatest opportunity for independence while the individual's changing needs can be monitored through the regular participation in the service program. This system is relatively easy to enter, because it requires no change of residence and the individual can quickly alter the intensity of services received, and is the least expensive way in which services can be provided.

The integrated home and service center model provides:

1. Primary setting in which services are offered:
   Senior Center or other health or recreational program
2. Services:
   Transportation
   Meals
   Health screening and clinics
   Recreation
   Education
   Hobbies
   Counseling
   Physical exercise
   Social and community action
   Employment
   Home chore services
   Home health care
   Day health care
   Housing renovation
   Legal services
   Telephone reassurance
   Shopping assistance

## The Congregate Service Model

The congregate service model differs from the integrated home–service center model in that a level of institutionalization has been introduced by the older person's living in a setting where certain supports are always at hand. A measure of independence is sacrificed for a more regular schedule of surveillance and supervision. The congregate service model generally offers some basic services in addition to housing and general supervision, including a meal, transportation, and some recreation. Here, however, the recreation is most frequently with the occupants of the same housing setting rather than with the larger community. The frail person gains additional services at the place of residence in exchange for reduced social opportunities.

The role of the family is lessened because the institution has assumed greater responsibilities for surveillance and supplying or calling for appropriate services as needed. Because of limited public commitment to this model, few congregate living arrangements have been established and those that exist have long waiting lists. It is obvious that a service that is unavailable or available only in the distant future is of no use to the older person, nor is there any immediate value in being placed on a long waiting list. There also is limited public support for the services immediately attached to the congregate service model (home health, counseling, housekeeping), and additional services have to be arranged on the basis of each person's eligibility for the service. Some effort has been made to develop small group homes having some of the qualities of the congregate living arrangements, but this too has had little public support. Major public policy changes will have to take place for congregate housing to be a viable alternative.

A new congregate service package has been introduced by the Department of Housing and Urban Development (HUD) on a demonstration basis, but its scope is too small at this time to expect it to have any immediate impact on the development of this model.

The congregate service model provides:

1. Primary settings in which services are offered:
   Foster homes
   Group homes
   Congregate apartments
   Homes for the aging
   Board and care homes
2. Services:
   Meals
   Recreation
   Education
   Hobbies
   General surveillance and supervision
   Housekeeping and chore service
   Health education and clinics
   Transportation
   Home health care
   Home chore services
   Shopping assistance

## The Home Care Model

The home care model differs from the integrated home–service center model by delivering services primarily to the individual at home. This model assumes a degree of frailty that prevents regular participation in programs outside the home. Essentially, the individual is homebound and on occasion may be bedridden. While this model is idealized because it enables an individual to avoid institutionalization and remain at home, it has severe limitations in the quantity of services that can be delivered to the home and its potential for social interactions. This model is not desirable for those who are bedridden, for whom its maintenance may provide limited services yet require the highest expenditure of money.

The level of surveillance is low in this model, and the older person spends most of the day alone unless a caretaker is present. Telephone assurance programs, visits by neighbors, and calls from family notwithstanding, most of the elderly person's time is spent alone. Although services like meals, homemaker assistance, and home health and chore services may be brought into the household on a regular basis, there may be no opportunity for social interactions with peers.

Family participation is extremely important, and requires a "living in" arrangement or regular visits for surveillance. Control or monitoring is generally low because of the difficulty of supervising home care. Funding for home care is sporadic, so that while food service is generally easy to provide, regular home health care is more difficult to justify, even though it may be the essential service to enable the person to remain at home.

The independence that makes this model so important may in fact be a vision of what had been or what possibly might recur. However, the frail person institutionalized at home may only have succeeded in exercising some degree of independence to select a less than desirable living arrangement. This option is sometimes viewed as undesirable from the service providers' point of view, because of the difficulty in delivering services. Despite these caveats, it may have significant value for some older persons who associate remaining independent with staying in their own homes. These people should be made aware of any other options to this model and shown how availability of services may alter their choice. For this model to be more effective, public support must assure the continuity of regular visits by a home health team or care providers.

The home care model provides:

1. Primary setting in which services are offered:
   Home

2. Services:
    Telephone assurance
    Homemaker
    Home health
    Meals and/or food
    Transportation to medical care

    Day health care
    Friendly visiting
    Shopping

## The Institutional Care Model

The institutional level of care should be reserved for persons in any of three following categories: those who cannot be maintained in any of the three levels of care described above; those who require this care for a period of rehabilitation or post–acute care restoration, but who will return to another level of residence within an expected time; or those who need institutionalization for brief periods of respite for themselves or for family care providers.

Institutional care has the highest level of surveillance and readily available services of any of the models described, but it may be accompanied by the lowest level of independence. It also requires the highest level of public support in terms of money made available and the greatest amount of public control, achieved through licensing and inspections. Public support of money and controls has not, however, assured consistently high levels of performance or of public confidence in this kind of service.

The institutional care model provides:

1. Primary setting in which services are offered:
    Skilled nursing facility
    Intermediate care facility
    Hospital extended-care units
2. Services:
    Room and board
    Nursing care
    Medical care
    Recreation
    Transportation
    Counseling
    Physical therapy
    Occupational therapy
    Religious services
    Social services

A review of the four models described above illustrates the range of potentials in the delivery of services. Today the older, chronically ill person does not have equal access to each of the models and therefore does not in fact have the opportunity to choose among them. While nursing home care may be viewed as an entitlement because of the relative ease of securing public payment for nursing home care, other levels of home care or congregate care are not readily available because adequate funds to generate those services are not available. The exercise of options among different levels of care cannot be realized until there is an assumed entitlement for reasonable services in each of these four models, with the funds available to provide the services.

## Administration

Important components of the long-term care system are its administrative arrangements and capacity to deliver the services, account for their use, make appropriate payments, and monitor and evaluate their effectiveness. These administrative functions should be separate from any of the organizations providing services, but could be included among the responsibilities for the core services described earlier. While most of the services identified will retain their autonomous ownership and management, participation in the system requires centralized entry, case management, data collection, and evaluation. The necessary administrative services, which will be discussed in subsequent chapters, include planning; fiscal accountability; data collection and reporting; program assessment and monitoring; manpower training and development; research; advocacy; and protective services—commitment, guardianship, conservatorship, and power of attorney.

Figure 1 summarizes the discussion dealing with components of long-term care, and correlates the proposed services with recommendations for sponsorship and funding. Administrative and core services for the coordinated long-term care system should be provided by a single community-wide organization having sole responsibility in an area currently within the planning jurisdiction of the health systems agency. Because the core services should be entitlements, funds should be provided directly to each organization, based on the number of persons in that planning area requiring services.

Services offered by the four models should be provided by individual public or private agencies, with funds coming from private sources, third party payers, or federal programs making payments for long-term care services. These service agencies need not revise their

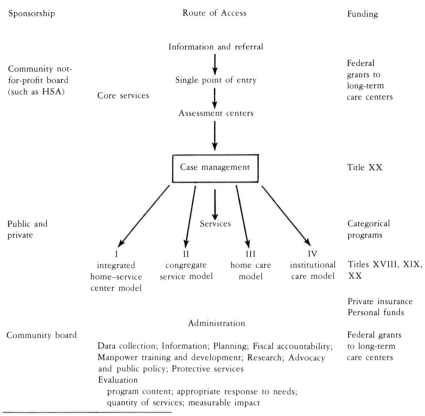

Fig. 1.   Components of Long-Term Care

current organizational structure or submerge their organization into the long-term care system. The system should permit providers to maintain their independence and specialization while making the providers of core services responsible for determining the best level of care for each participant. Improving the effectiveness of the entire system should be a funded part of the core services.

## Summary

About two to three million older people, or 12 percent to 14 percent of the population sixty-five years of age and over, suffer from the impairments of chronic illness yet live in their own homes. This is in addition to the more than 1.25 million, or about 5 percent of this population, who reside in nursing homes.

Long-term care is not defined by the length of time that

services are provided but rather by the extent of chronicity of the illness. Thus, about three million older persons are in need of long-term care services because of the presence of chronic illness and its disabilities. The older person should have a choice of available services that permit remaining at home when feasible. A continuum of care should be made available and should include a close union of related parts of a system, including services offered at home, in nonresidential service centers, in congregate housing programs, and in institutional facilities. Core services, or those services essential to maintaining the network of services, also need to be incorporated and should be entitlements of those who are chronically ill. These include information, referral, outreach, assessment, and case management. Additionally, administrative services, education, and evaluation should be available to assure the successful operation of the long-term care program.

# Chapter
# 5

# Organization
# of the
# Long-Term Care
# System

*. . . [L]ong-term care refers to health and social services provided to
chronically disabled, usually elderly persons. . . . efforts to ensure that
older persons are placed at appropriate levels of care have been plagued
by fragmentation of responsibility and by lack of adequate placement
criteria and assessment mechanisms. In general, the elderly face a
bewildering collection of fragmented long-term care services and
financing arrangements.*

*. . . [T]he elderly who are the most vulnerable to the loss of
their ability to "maintain independence and dignity in a home
environment" are those whose chronic impairments have become disabling. Most are of advanced age, seventy-five years and older. Their
circumstances are often exacerbated by low income, the absence of
family, and isolation from a community support system.*

LONG-TERM CARE GERONTOLOGY CENTER GUIDELINES,
ADMINISTRATION ON AGING

## The Environment of Long-Term Care

Institutional and noninstitutional programs are often
viewed as being in an adversary relationship in which the home and
the institution compete to be considered the best provider of long-
term care. Services delivered in the home frequently are described as
*the* community care system, as if that system did not also include
health care institutions. It can be argued, however, that the long-

term care system ideally includes the full range of services available to the person with chronic illness and this includes the institution. The preference of older people is typically to remain at home, especially if an assessment indicates that they can do so if certain services are provided. That preference must be weighed against the economic and other advantages of congregating services at a central location.

A useful approach to the issue of the most suitable site for providing services is Lawton's "ecological change model" (1974). This model argues "that desirable responses may be elicited, or elevated in quality, by the provision of a favorable environment. . . . [T]he hypothesis suggests that methods which directly increase the competence of the individual will give him greater control over his environment. The model looks at treatment in terms of whether the measures are applied to the individual or to the environment, and whether the individual initiates the treatment or responds to the external application of the treatment."

This model suggests that the most positive growth can occur when people make their own decisions about what help will be most useful in overcoming some of the disabilities of chronic illness. Creative changes in the living environment, when they are responsive to the needs of older people, can improve their competence and confidence: "A change in environment will be most effective in changing behavior when the individual is at a threshold level of competence." Stated another way, "the payoff for effective environmental intervention is very high for older people in poor mental or physical health" (Lawton 1974).

Effective environmental changes range from such responses to sensory losses as improved lighting, sound or visual clues, (see Ernst and Shore 1975 for a thorough discussion of sensory losses), to entire environments designed for older people (see Koncelik 1976; and Lawton, Newcomer, and Byerts 1976). Other environmental changes may introduce older people to new social relationships and support structures, giving them opportunities to feel good about themselves when the family's involvement in care is occasional and minimal. On the other hand, the absence of a direct caring role creates problems for some children or relatives who want to be more actively involved in the care program and therefore environmental design should permit family involvement.

In the context of the continuum of services, described in an earlier chapter, there are no alternatives to institutional care; institutions must remain as an important part of the continuum. There are two additional models which represent modifications to the home model versus institution model paradigm. The options of the integrated home-service center model, congregate service model, home care model and institutional model permit options for care delivery that can directly increase the competence of older people to deal with problems of chronic illnesses. This conceptualization is far preferable to the home-institution dichotomy. The full range of levels of care, viewed as a system, provides multiple opportunities for modifying living arrangements to accommodate to changing needs of older people.

## Administering the System

In its report, *The Future of Long Term Care in the United States,* the National Conference on Social Welfare (1977) identified a number of issues it called "dilemmas" in the evolving long-term care system. The primary one of these was, "where should administrative authority for long-term care be located?" The possibilities are the health system or the social services system.

The Arden House Institute on Continuity of Long-Term Care (1977) argued that "there should be a state plan and a state level policy unit with continuing responsibility to prepare such a plan and to correlate the work of necessary participant agencies." An examination of some of the successful long-term care programs reveals that they have either public or private sponsoring organizations, and are principally a product of local community efforts. In the absence of either a major national policy on long-term care or specific guidelines for developing coordinated long-term care programs, the creativity of local efforts is even more noteworthy. Where programs have been designed by the local community and successfully evolved from the unique character of the local community and its service composition, it should be maintained. The sponsoring agency for the long-term care program has generally been aided through federal grants to design the system and to provide the core services—usually including administration, assessment, and case management—while the direct service agencies retain their own functional autonomy. Some process, generally described as purchase of service, is then used to acquire the necessary service components for each individual.

The following recommendations outline a long-term care system that would encompass the existing health and social service programs (see figure 2):

1. A long-term care system agency should be established and designated the community agency to coordinate and develop long-term care services. The areas already designated for Health Systems Agencies (HSA's) could be designated as service areas for a long-term care system. This designation would recognize the HSA area as a long-term care planning area.

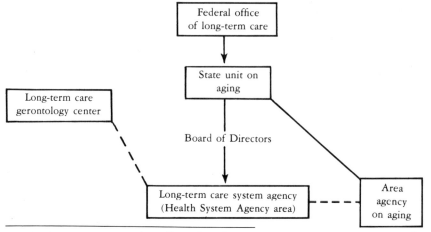

**Fig. 2.**   Organization of the Long-Term Care System

Where area agencies on aging exist, they should be integrated into the planning, if not designated the primary planning agency for long-term care.

2. The federal government should provide direct funding to the long-term care system agency, based on the numbers of persons over age seventy-five currently residing in the designated area (seventy-five is an arbitrary figure, but around that age incidence of chronic illness increases alarmingly). This funding should be used for administration of the agency and the provision of core (information, referral, outreach, assessment centers, case management, and administrative) services—which then would become an entitlement for all persons seventy-five years and older (See *Public Policy and the Frail Elderly* 1978). While the emphasis is on those age seventy-five and older, the long-term care program should be responsive to younger chronically ill persons in need of services.

3. The new long-term care system agency should not integrate itself into the existing health or social services systems, but should align itself with any agencies whose goals are compatible with those of the long-term care agency and its services, representing a multidisciplinary approach.

4. Under permissive guidelines promulgated by the federal government a local, private, nonprofit board of directors should be constituted to assume responsibility for the new agency in order to be approved for funding. The composition of the board should be appropriate to the local community and its previous efforts in providing long-term care services. The board should adopt a statement of philosophy and goals for the long-term care services.

5. The new long-term care agency should have clearly identified collaborative relationships with the Health Systems Agency

to assure orderly growth, licensing, and funding for long-term care services essential to support the total long-term care system in each community.

6. The federal government should designate an office of long-term-care to coordinate the efforts of the local agencies. In addition, a national council on long-term care should also be established to provide direction and support to the federal office of long-term care and promote public policies in support of the long-term care system.

7. The state unit on aging should coordinate all of the individual long-term care agencies to prevent overlapping services, to encourage the statewide development of agencies, and to coordinate the long-term care agencies with other research, demonstrations, or educational programs in each state.

8. Each long-term care system should be related to one of the long-term care gerontology centers and programs of research; education and new model development should be coordinated between the agency and the center.

The core of the long-term care services agencies could be built upon existing long-term care demonstrations where they have been established, and their continuity could be supported by additional resources as needed. Development of like agencies in other communities should be encouraged, to assure a greater distribution of long-term care systems throughout the country. A federal commitment to fund long-term care agencies would establish a much needed public policy in support of long-term care as a united, comprehensive system of services for older people with debilitating chronic illnesses.

# Major Units in the Core System

Kammerman and Kahn (1976) point out that any system which delivers services to clients needs to provide for access, integration, and accountability. These issues are highlighted in the discussion that follows. In that special system referred to as long-term care, these issues are of special importance because the clients are often frail and therefore not capable of asserting themselves in a complicated health and social service system. The client must gain access to the services, the services have to be administered so that they are responsive to the client's needs, and the services must be delivered to each client.

Getting people into the long-term care system at the right time is critical to the successful delivery of the appropriate services. It requires changed behavior on the part of the care providers who usually refer older people for service—physicians, hospital discharge planners, social agencies, and so on. The presence of the coordinated system, its value to the individual older person and community, and its appropriate use must be interpreted to each new client. This is especially critical where the long-term care system represents a major change in the way services have been negotiated in the past.

Chapter 4 presented an outline of the essential services in long-term care and the process for introducing the services. These will now be described in greater detail.

## Information, Outreach, and Referral

It is essential that the community know about the developing long-term care services, how the services are administered, and how applications are processed.

Three levels of public information must be addressed. The first requires that specific information be available to providers of services and those who refer clients for service. This could take the form of written brochures, forums for the care providers, and/or personal contacts with providers.

Second, information should be processed through organizations of older people or programs specifically serving the older person, such as senior centers or senior nutrition sites, or through physicians' offices. Both of these approaches can be reinforced by general announcements in the press, radio, and television.

The most difficult part of this task is outreach, which attempts to locate the frail older person living alone or in an isolated lifestyle. This person may not be in contact with any of the health or social agencies. If people appear to *want* to be out of reach of the community's health service system, do we have the right to reach out and urge their use of long-term care services? Certainly we do, but such intervention must be accompanied by respect for the right of the individual to refuse any or all of the proffered services.

Isolated individuals might be found through referrals by other older persons, neighbors, or members of other service networks, such as the mail carriers. A special telephone number for an information and referral service, well advertised as a resource for older persons, also could be valuable.

It is important to note that the older person living alone may be fearful of the inquiring community worker because conventional wisdom suggests that involvement by social agency representatives generally results in institutionalization. "There is no question that older people would prefer to remain in their homes in the community rather than go to an institution. . . . It is clear that a large number of older people would choose the stress and possible deprivation of living independently rather than accept the security and control of life in an institution" (Lawton 1978). It will often take considerable effort to convince cautious or distrustful older people that appropriate intervention could improve their lives without necessarily resorting to institutional placement.

## Assessment

The major resources of the coordinated long-term care system are the process of assessment and its use as the single point of entry into the system. The assessment, based on a diagnosis of the individual's health condition, as well as an evaluation of the social systems and the environment, attempts to relate the most appropriate package of services to the needs of the individual.

The single point of entry tries to assure that assessment will actually lead to access to services. Single point of entry also means that once a person enters the system, that person need not go through the assessment process every time there is a change in functional capacity—although there may be need for a multidisciplinary review or update of any part of the assessment. It also means the person need not reapply for other levels of services in the system although changes occur. Once in the system, the person is referred to services determined by the assessment team.

The assessment process at the single point of entry should be the only way a person can be assigned to a case manager and the appropriate programs. This means that no one gains access to services in the coordinated system without an assessment having been made.

The assessment team may elect to omit any part of the complete assessment process, based on observable behavior or recently completed physical assessment in a hospital.

Ishizaki, Gottesman, and McBride (1979) described two models for service management as central intake and multiple access with central responsibility. Central intake is a system in which all clients enter through one central agency. Central intake assumes that involved providers will accept assessments and case plans prepared by the intake unit, and will provide services as prescribed.

Multiple access with central responsibility is a system in which clients can enter a coordinated community service network by way of any one of several major cooperating service providers. An assessment is done by one of the cooperating providers and a service plan is written. The client is then referred to other providers when additional services are required, but no agency provides intake for another.

A combination of the two models described above is possible when multiple access sites make it possible for any one of them to provide intake for participants. Care remains a central responsibility, regardless of the site of assessment or site of entry into the system. Because the assessment center is not likely to replace all other forms of intake or assessment soon, the option for some people to apply directly to a service provider should be continued. Obviously some private agencies may elect to remain outside the long-term care system, providing their services without public support or intervention. While this option must remain, the obvious value of the use of the assessment center and single point of entry should be demonstrated to both agencies and older people who use the system. Obviously, the more comprehensive the program, i.e., its inclusion of the largest possible number of long-term care services in the community, the more effective it can be in providing a choice of services.

The ultimate goal of assessment and the single point of entry is to provide the most appropriate array of services to each older person at the lowest cost. The Triage Program (1975) of Rochester, New York, elaborates on this theme and lists six objectives, which include: providing a single entry mechanism by which the elderly can have their physical, social, psychological, and life-support needs evaluated; developing, through demonstrated need, necessary preventive and supportive services; integrating the efforts of service providers to give coordinated care; creating financial support as needed for the full spectrum of services; demonstrating by documentation the value of basic preventive and supportive services; demonstrating the cost-effectiveness of coordinated care.

Agencies that remain outside the system may inflate the cost of care and, therefore, public expense when the absence of appropriate assessment results in use of higher levels of care or a more costly service than is necessary. The reward for the older person and society at large should be provision of the most appropriate care at the lowest possible cost. The administration of an individual program should be rewarded by making it possible for it to maintain its income adequately in spite of reduced occupancy caused by the changed referral policies. Preserving the economic security of component agencies requires close cooperative planning among the long-term care agency, the health systems agency, and the funding agencies for health and social service.

*The Assessment Center*

Designing an appropriate service system for elderly persons depends upon knowing the impairments of each individual as well as identifying residual capacities and potential for gaining new knowledge and skills. The comprehensive evaluation of the individual should assess more than health status. The range of problems experienced by older people and the services that are required extend well beyond health problems and health services. They include mental health problems and services, social and economic problems and services, and impairments in capacity for self-care, along with services aimed at supplementing or restoring self-care capacity. Moreover, each of these areas of functioning influences other areas of functioning, for better or for worse.

Pfeiffer (1973) stresses the interrelationship of problems influencing the total functioning capacity of the individual. He also cautions that practitioners without special training in working with the aged tend to reach premature judgments regarding their overall functioning, and tend to discover problems related to the practitioner's area of specialization. The importance of appropriate training of the assessment team and the use of a multidisciplinary team are, therefore, critical.

Lawton and Brody (1969) view human behavior as related to the complexity of functioning required by a variety of living tasks. The lowest level is called life maintenance, followed by successively more complex levels such as functional health, and ultimately, social behavior. Each level of functioning generally requires greater complexity of neuropsychological organization than the one preceding it. The individual is "assessed by measuring instruments designed to tap representative behavior at each level and within the range of competence appropriate to the individual." The assessment should, of course, include the clinical assessment of psychological functioning as part of the comprehensive assessment approach.

Many assessment instruments have been developed to assist and systematize observations about the degree of impairment and functioning of potential recipients of long-term care. The Federal Council on Aging (1978) reviewed seventeen assessment instruments analyzed in an HEW study, and recommended the "Physical Self-Maintenance Scale and Instrumental Activities of Daily Living," developed by Lawton and Brody at the Philadelphia Geriatric Center and "The OARS Methodology," developed by the Duke Center for the Study of Aging and Human Development as most applicable to a multidimensional approach to assessing the frail elderly. According to Lawton and Brody (1969):

> It is generally accepted that assessment of older people is a complex process requiring evaluation from different vantage points. The notable lack of preventive services and the scarcity of resources compound the difficulties since planning often must take place at a time when the capacities of the elderly

person are clouded by acute reality problems and the emotional upset of elderly individuals and family members. Measures which compel focused attention to the functioning of the older person are therefore important tools in any attempt to bring order to the planning process.

Instruments used in assessment should be part of an over-all systematic approach, should be adaptable to varied settings and goals, and should foster communication between the related professionals and agencies. Because the assessment process should attempt to obtain an accurate understanding of the person's capacities to function in the basic activities of daily living as well as in social relationships, it is important that assessments be performed in social settings that reflect as closely as possible the real living challenges faced by the older person. Some aspect of the assessment should be conducted in the person's home. The adult day care center might be an appropriate assessment site.

The process of assessment should also include a systematized evaluation of the environment, quantified through the use of an environmental assessment instrument. Unfortunately, the technology of environmental assessment is not yet as sophisticated as that of the individual assessment. When the two assessment processes (individual and environmental) can be coordinated, it may be possible to devise a correlation matrix to determine what characteristics of the environment are necessary to compensate for losses in functional capacities.

## Case Management

Finding appropriate resources for human services is difficult in any community. For the frail elderly person, or his or her surrogate, seeking services that will respond quickly to critical living problems is at best very difficult. The effectiveness of the long-term care system in providing appropriate services at the right time is dependent upon the case manager (sometimes called facilitator).

The difficulty of locating services may then be compounded by the processes for determining eligibility and certifying an individual for a particular service. Case management is necessary because many older persons "fall between the cracks," or are ineligible for appropriate use of existing resources. Case management is an important part of the integrated approach. It attempts to select the most appropriate level of service for each individual and provides the transition point between the assessment process and the effective delivery of service.

Case management is defined by Access (1979) as an "administrative service defined as the management of a process that includes the coordination of a comprehensive preadmission assessment, the development of a service plan, the initiation of home services or placement assistance, and follow-up monitoring. The main objective is to assure ongoing delivery of the right care in the right amount in a timely and cost-effective manner."

In the Access system the case manager performs the following functions: screens referrals for service; coordinates the assessment (including medical, nursing, and psychosocial evaluation, physician consultation and work-up, financial counseling, home assessments, and social work assessment; assures client consent to participate; certifies necessity for a specific level of care; assures client notification of potential for home care; optimizes client choice in care plan selection; assures medical eligibility; approves Medicaid payments; supervises the initiation of the care plan; assures continuity of care; and monitors change in the client's service needs.

From another point of view, case management functions are described by Callahan (1979) to include the following: making collaborative arrangements to assure continuity of services regardless of the auspices of the provider; making necessary care arrangements; referring to appropriate service and coordinating its delivery; arranging for covered items and services; maintaining a continuous relationship with the individual; acting as a service broker by matching individual needs and resources; and insuring delivery of services.

Because older people using the long-term care services generally have multiple problems, they often find it necessary to have contact with more than one provider at a time. Also, just as the needs of the older person are continuous, so is the need for case management.

Advocacy on behalf of the client is an inherent part of case management as the staff member seeks the appropriate service, the funds to provide the service, and assurance that the older person will benefit from the service provided. It is the case manager who will request changes in the level or kind of service, or a reassessment for the older person.

The presence of supporting family members may or may not preclude the need for a case management service. Family members may not be adequately versed in services, eligibility, or responses to changing needs, and may benefit from the supports offered by the case management approach. The availability of case management should not suggest that family members are superfluous.

## Providing Access to Services

The assessment process should have as one of its products a written prescription of services required by each individual. It is important that the assessment process be an educational experience for the older person and the family, so each step should be noted in the records and explained to the client and his or her family. Another important product of assessment is the initiation of a data collection system, to be discussed later.

Access to services probably could be accomplished through any combination of three procedures, depending upon available payments or services. The first is to arrange for services based upon the individual's current eligibility, where this eligibility is clearly determined as entitlement. The second is to purchase services for the client from funds available to the long-term care program. These funds may be available for special demonstration programs or as waivers to eligibility. The third is to stimulate the development of new services or modifications of existing services to meet needs that have become evident through the assessment process. It is in this area that cooperative action with health systems agencies becomes critical, because the relationship is used to further develop needed services as well as to identify funds appropriate for the new service. The potential for upgrading services through innovative changes argues for placing the long-term care agency in juxtaposition to the health systems agency if the agency continues its function of health services planning.

## Data Systems

The ability of the managers of the long-term care program to plan for their clients' needs is dependent in part on their ability to gather and assess information related to current services, including data on what should be available as well as what is. Developing an adequate data system requires a clear statement of the purposes of the long-term care services. The long-term care program should be concerned with issues of morbidity and mortality of the older persons, as well as with maintenance of a quality of life in which the individual's dignity and opportunity for choice of lifestyle are enhanced. Other goals of the program should relate to reduced use of acute care services, maintenance of a satisfactory health status, and a person's ability to handle activities of daily living, continuation of socialization, and heightened consumer satisfaction. Data gathered and their subsequent examination should provide answers to questions that deal with the ability of the long-term care program to meet its objectives.

Data should be accessible to concerned professionals beginning with the assessment process, when the multidimensional assessment of each applicant for service establishes initial baseline information. Information dealing with physical and mental health, social functioning, economic resources, and functional strengths and impairments is gathered during the assessment process and determines what services may be required. This information, stored and used to follow and evaluate the progress of each participant, can provide cumulative information that will enable the analyst better to understand and evaluate the total long-term care service system.

Furthermore, comparisons among several long-term care systems or any national effort to develop data on long-term care depend upon having each long-term care service system participate in the collection of comparable data. The federal government could lead the way in establishing uniform recordkeeping, cost accounting, and tracking systems. This would require the use of comparable assessment instruments and data collection among the varied participants. Common training should be provided participants in each program, and the cost of data collection should be underwritten through a specified budget, funded by the federal government as part of its support of core services. The data processes should not be paid for from service funds, but should instead be supported by funds specifically designated for data systems thus indicating commitment to a national coordinated data collection program. The rewards to each program for participation in the national effort, beyond the sharing of funding resources, should include the availability of frequently distributed composite reports of all participants, accompanied by analysis of commonalities, departures from common experiences, and observable trends in services. These reports, collected over a period of time, would become valuable tools for influencing national and local public policies, and would have the potential to serve as the basis for constructive planning in long-term care.

A basic input-output system for long-term care has been suggested by Callahan (1979) and is illustrated in figure 3. Variables selected for use in this schema come from *Long-Term Care: Minimum Data Set,* U.S. National Committee on Vital and Health Statistics (1978). The data set defines a central core of data about a given dimension of health and health services needed on a routine basis by the majority of users, as well as standardized measurements and classifications. This data set could be adapted to form the core of a long-term care data system, and enlarged or modified as subsequent use might dictate.

In addition to identifying the characteristics of the service needs of clients through the use of this minimum data set, the long-term care data system should elicit information that will answer questions that deal with the number of programs providing services in the four service models described earlier. Details related to services provided, costs of providing services, and sources for funding of services should be stored in the system and be easily retrievable.

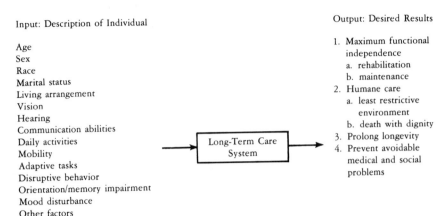

Input: Description of Individual

Output: Desired Results

Age
Sex
Race
Marital status
Living arrangement
Vision
Hearing
Communication abilities
Daily activities
Mobility
Adaptive tasks
Disruptive behavior
Orientation/memory impairment
Mood disturbance
Other factors

Long-Term Care
System

1. Maximum functional
   independence
   a. rehabilitation
   b. maintenance
2. Humane care
   a. least restrictive
      environment
   b. death with dignity
3. Prolong longevity
4. Prevent avoidable
   medical and social
   problems

*Source:* Adapted from J. J. Callihan, "The Organization of The Long-Term Care System and the Potential for a Single Agency Option" (Ph.D. diss., Brandeis University, 1979).

**Fig. 3.**  Long-Term Care System: Input-Output Overview

The process of evolving a comprehensive network of long-term care services requires that information relating to composite group data and service trends be treated as equal in importance to data dealing with the individual participants' service needs and use of the system. Coordination of the two types of information would create a comprehensive resource for understanding and improving the nation's ability to meet the needs of its chronically ill older people. Strategies for making an impact on policy changes is dependent upon the availability of data describing the programs and their impact.

The availability of specific data is also essential for the evaluation of long-term care programs. "Health professionals have long agreed that consistently good care is tied to consistently good performance and is not accidental, but rather the result of a systematic process." (Miller and Knapp 1979). If the long-term care system is eventually to be more effective than the efforts of earlier unrelated service agencies providing care for the chronically ill, it is incumbent upon the long-term care organization to give evidence of improved care.

Tomlinson, Trager, and Cohen (1976) suggest four areas of long-term care that require careful attention to improve the care. The first of these is *quality,* or the ability of both individuals and organizations to deliver the care the group is expected to provide. For example, the quality of care provided by an institution, or home care, or any aspect of service such as the home-delivered meals program, must be made objectively measurable. Although many methods for evaluating the quality of care programs have been advanced, no universally accepted comprehensive approach is yet available. Obviously it is more difficult to evaluate the complicated nature of institutional care than it is to measure the quality of a meal service to someone who is homebound. Some professional organizations (American Nurses Association, the National League for Nursing, the National Association of Social Workers, the National Association of Homemaker–Home Health Aide Services) have defined quality, and have suggested quality standards and guidelines (Tomlinson, Trager, and Cohen 1976). Their having done so implies that each profession can establish its own standards and advance a system to monitor the professionals' adherence to the standard. Three major approaches for evaluating the quality of care are commonly used today. They are the organizational assessment, in which staffing, facilities, and procedures are examined; the outcome assessment, in which a person's state of health or functional capacity is measured after services are provided; and the process assessment, in which the quantity of care given to the client is the focus of inquiry (Miller and Knapp 1979). The assessment may be done by an outside voluntary organization, such as the Joint Commission on Accreditation of Hospitals and any of its subunits that accredit other levels of health care; by the Professional Standards Review Organization, mandated by federal legislation in PL92-603, Social Security Act Amendments of 1972; by peer review of an identified professional group; or by multidisciplinary peer group assessment committees. The latter is recommended, since the multidisciplinary nature of long-term care services requires that outcome or process evaluations of the organizational objectives be viewed from the perspective of the varied professional disciplines provided in a comprehensive service package. The reorganization of typical service roles by single disciplines, essential to providing total care for those with chronic illnesses, requires that assessment methodologies be made compatible with the manner in which services are to be delivered.

The quality assessment process should include the use of a multidisciplinary peer group structure which should involve, in addition to representatives of the chronically ill who depend upon some aspects of the long-term care system for their support, families of those who use the system and, where available, representatives of an ombudsman's office or other advocacy groups. The quality of long-term care is too important to be viewed as the exclusive province of any one professional group or as the sole responsibility of the professions involved in the delivery of long-term care. Appropriate representation from consumers, advocates, and public officials should insure that the quest for quality care be understood as a shared goal and therefore a shared, mutual responsibility of major segments of the care providers, recipients of care, public officials, and funding resources.

The second aspect of evaluation to be considered is *appropriateness,* which attempts to match the service (in terms of kind, mix, quantity, and timing) to the need by referring the older person to the proper agency to receive care. One of the underlying reasons for developing the system of long-term care is that services provided independently of others often result in care that is either too much, too little, or of the wrong kind. It has been suggested earlier that an applicant for institutional care is probably evaluated differently depending on whether or not the institution has a waiting list or empty beds. The long-term care system should be so organized as to avoid determination of need for services that is based on the needs of the service provider rather than the needs of the older person. The problem of appropriateness is compounded when services must be selected from inappropriate alternatives.

The third issue is *equity,* which requires agreement to adhere to quality and appropriateness standards, eligibility requirements, service availability, and ease of access to care so that all individuals with like needs receive like care. Even when a full range of services of equal quality is offered in an area as a whole, there may be inequity for some older people because access to services is the product of geography. This is especially true where urban-rural differences are related to the availability of financial resources to purchase services.

The fourth issue is *cost-effectiveness,* or the meeting of well-defined objectives at the least possible cost. This important issue is difficult to measure because of the lack of clearly defined objectives. This limitation can be overcome, however, and the goal of developing cost-effective measures should be sustained. It would be valuable to understand the impact of underuse or overuse of services on the cost of providing care, as well as to determine the costs generated by the inequities of geography or eligibility requirements. It is possible that appropriate use of services would prove to be cost-efficient because of the reduced need for more costly services, even though the array of services made available would undoubtedly increase the total cost for the system because of the larger number of people served. On the other hand, efforts toward cost containment or restriction of use by regulations related to deductibles or coinsurance may be costly because they may allow chronic conditions to deteriorate until they require more costly services or greater intensity of services. Such outcomes increase both the eventual cost for services and the burden for the person who is chronically ill.

## Funding

Having dealt with the important characteristics of the system's core services, or those features that differentiate the coordinated long-term care system from an array of uncoordinated autonomous services, it is important to examine some of the contemporary issues related to the funding of long-term care. Both the services identified in the system and the delivery of any of those services are subject to major modification—especially in a rapidly evolving long-term care system—but the most critical of all the many aspects subject to major modification is funding. This is so because the primary source of funding for all long-term care systems in the United States is the federal government, and funding is therefore subject to its changing priorities. Any of the systems proposed or services necessary to enable such systems to function are dependent upon the continuity of funds. Continued funding, in turn, depends on the expectations of the funding agencies or of Congress. Unfortunately, the federal government has made no clear commitment to sustain funding for a comprehensive long-term care system.

Yet there is ample reason to believe that changes have to be made in the way our society responds to the needs of chronically ill older people, and that the federal government is prepared to invest in demonstration or exploratory programs to learn how to provide better services. Uncertainty about the continuity of funding after successful demonstrations makes urgent the need for public policy changes that would assure an ongoing commitment to the long-term care system.

In addition to the funded demonstrations of community care systems by the Administration on Aging and the Health Care Financing Administration, the Administration on Aging has initiated a new program to develop long-term care gerontology centers throughout the nation. These are proposed as university programs involving medical schools, other schools of related health services and community services, and community service systems for the chronically ill aged, joined together to form centers for research, education, and service. It is anticipated that these centers will become permanent parts of university organizations and serve as focal points for new community thrusts toward improving the nation's response to the increasing needs of the older population.

At the same time, the United States Department of Health and Human Services (DHHS) has initiated a program involving the Health Care Financing Administration, the Administration on Aging, and the Public Health Service, and coordinated by the Assistant Secretary for Planning and Evaluation, which is described as a National Long-Term Care Channeling Agency Demonstration Program. This program is ". . . designed to test the extent to which a local structure to manage and coordinate in-home, community based, and institutional long-term care services will assure that people who need long-term care receive the appropriate types and levels of services in a more efficient and cost-effective manner. The principal target population for the Channeling Agency Demonstration Program will be functionally impaired elderly" (HEW Memorandum 1979).

HHS recognizes that long-term care, with its current emphasis on institutional care, is placing a major strain on federal, state, and local public financing. New approaches will have to be devised to respond to the increasing needs of the rapidly growing older population.

*Channeling* is defined as a mechanism for appropriately linking clients to needed types and levels of services to result in more effective, cost efficient, and humane policies and programs. These demonstration programs have been designed to test innovative approaches to the organization, financing, and delivery of long-term care services, to gather national baseline data to evaluate the program, and to recommend public policies in support of effective approaches that will overcome some of the critical barriers to effective long-term care delivery.

Channeling agencies will be responsible for determining eligibility for channeling agency services; assessing client needs; developing plans of care that match services with needs, taking into account and encouraging informal supports; arranging for the necessary services for clients, and coordinating the delivery of services; monitoring the provision of services; and reassessing clients' needs periodically.

The federal government's most recent plans—the long-term care gerontology centers and the channeling agencies—give evidence of increased support for long-term care. The acid test will be the ongoing commitment of new federal dollars for the core services—identified partially by the expectations of the channeling agencies—and support of the services from existing program funds. The flow of funds will have to be supportive of the full network of services rather than favoring any one segment of the network.

Figure 4 illustrates the current status of multiple sources of funds and overlapping jurisdictions related to funding and administration of long-term care programs. The organization of long-term care should permit the emergence of creative local programs based on the unique characteristics of the community, the pooling of funds from a variety of resources, and the basic funding for core services met by the federal government. It should be evident from a study of figure 4 that pooling of funds is essential to support the variety of services in long-term care. Omitted from this schema are the sources of demonstration funds and resources for funding of the core services that currently fall outside the typical funding flow. These are illustrated in figure 5.

Contrary to its appearance, figure 4 is not presented to

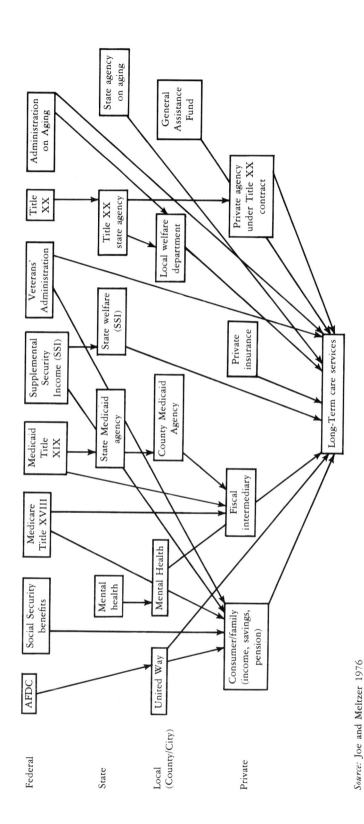

*Source:* Joe and Meltzer 1976

**Fig. 4.** Flow of Funds for Long-Term Care

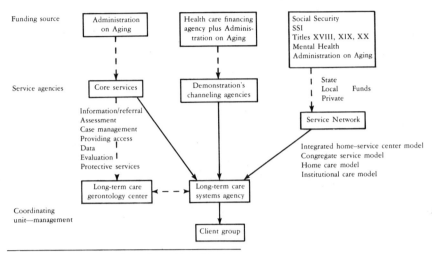

Fig. 5.   A Coordinated Long-Term Care Program

confuse the issue of funding, but rather to illustrate the importance of pooling resources and the confusion created by multiple funding sources. What this representation does not make clear are the priorities each funding source gives to long-term care. For example, the boxes representing funding sources should be drawn in sizes relative to the amount of their support, modified to show relative support for subunits of long-term care—i.e., monies for institutional care versus those for noninstitutional care. Ideally, the figure should be done in a form that would permit the various components to be enlarged (or more likely reduced) in size as public agencies modify funding of some aspects of a program. Because of limited resources, it is unlikely that there will be adequate increases in funding to respond to increased needs of those who are chronically ill.

The issues of funding for long-term care have to be dealt with on a broad policy level if adequate support, continuity of funding beyond demonstration phases, and the equity of funding distributed throughout the long-term care continuum are to be assured. If the federal government funds core services directly, this will establish access to assessment and all of the core services as an entitlement of the chronically ill older person.

However, the funding of individual services actually determines whether or not an older person can depend upon a particular service as part of a package. The complexity of existing eligibility requirements and multiple sources of funding argue for the preparation of a funding plan when the prescription for services is developed in the assessment phase. It is obvious that the mere presence of a service does not assure its availability to any client. Case managers must understand and be able to negotiate eligibility requirements in order to assure that the prescribed services are accessible to a given client.

In an era when the cost of health case services, and especially long-term care, are rising rapidly and the federal government seems intent on reducing federal expenditures for health care, new approaches for funding long-term care must be explored. Regulations and controls have been introduced to prevent use of unneeded services and to maintain limits on expenditures: "Utilization review committees, professional standards review organizations, and state personnel are required to review on a regular basis the appropriateness of institutional long-term care services. The costs to the public sector of these reviews have not been well documented, but they appear to be substantial. The effectiveness of these review processes in preventing inappropriate consumption of services can be questioned, as is shown by the large proportions of residents believed to be misplaced" (Win and McCaffree 1979).

Winn and McCaffree go on to say that the use of a prepaid capitation plan should be explored as an "alternative method for financing long-term care services which could integrate the financing of services presently provided by a variety of federal and state agencies." Capitation is a method of payment through which a fixed amount is paid on a regular basis without regard to the quantity of services used. Capitation plans are usually associated with health maintenance organizations, and have been used in some residential communities for older people (Scitovsky and Snyder 1970) and in demonstration projects of community care systems. Health maintenance organizations generally do not offer extensive long-term care services in their programs: "For example, only one-third of eighteen HMO arrangements offered any extended care benefits; in all cases this benefit was of limited duration, less than four months. Other benefits, such as services in the home, are similarly limited; although some plans offer these services for a limited period of time to help persons adjust after hospitalization, they are generally not available on a long-term basis" (Winn and McCaffree 1979).

Currently, prepaid health care plans do not enroll persons over sixty-five years of age unless they were former subscribers or are currently covered in an employee program.

Winn and McCaffree assume that a capitation system for long-term care will probably have the following characteristics: greater availability and enrollee use of alternatives to inpatient long-term care; lower enrollee use of inpatient services, as long as preventive services at home or other services reduce per capita costs; greater emphasis on services to maintain function and retard deterioration; and greater continuity of care.

These are all goals that are difficult to achieve in the

current fee-for-service arrangements but are part of the expected services of a long-term care system.

There is and should be public concern about the costs of long-term care, and especially the rapid escalation of costs. Rapidly rising costs have resulted from inflation, increased demands for services, and increasing numbers of older people who need services because of the problems related to chronic illness (Doherty and Hicks 1977; Volk, Hutchins, and Doremus 1980; Fox and Clauser, 1980; U.S. Dept. HEW, Health Care Financing Administration, 1981). The costs of nursing home care have been the fastest-rising component of personal health care expenditures. There are at this time conflicting reports regarding the possibility of reducing overall costs by substituting programs for nursing home care. Studies by Greenberg (1974) and Brickner (1980) suggest that money could be saved if some persons currently served in nursing homes were cared for at home. Brickner reports that home care programs for the frail homebound person cost three-fifths as much as the cost of nursing home care.

Weissert and others (1980) found that in a study of day care and home health services the cost for providing these services exceeded the cost of nursing home care. In an effort to assist in comparing costs of institutional and noninstitutional care, Doherty and Hicks (1977) distinguish between cost-effectiveness analysis and cost-benefit analysis. Cost-effectiveness is described as

> a technique for assessing and comparing the costs and effectiveness of alternative systems or programs; it is designed to assist decision makers in identifying a preferred choice or choices. Its contribution to the decision process is that it provides information and an analytical framework by which conclusions can be reached in a systematic and traceable way. . . . In cost-benefit analysis, both benefits and costs are typically reduced to monetary terms. In cost-effectiveness analysis, however, effectiveness need not be so reduced. The primary reason for the distinction is that it is not always useful or meaningful to aggregate program benefits or effects into economic indicators, be they utility or money.

In cost-effectiveness analysis the outcome is expressed in terms of effectiveness, or

> the extent to which alternative actions or programs accomplish their objectives. The difficulty however lies in the ability to specify effectiveness criteria in long-term care. . . . Undertaking a cost-effectiveness study requires that there be definable program goals (e.g., desirable health outcomes), alternative means

of attaining the goals (the programs to be compared), and constraints on the programs (the value of available resources). These prerequisites imply three steps to be taken: The programs to be compared must be identified as appropriate alternatives; the dimensions of program outcomes (both cost and effect) that are to be evaluated must be specified; and the technique to be used in the analysis must be described. (Doherty and Hicks 1977)

It is also important to note that expenditures for care do not necessarily equal the costs of producing that care: "Thus it is important to decide whether the economic outcome to be compared should relate to production or expenditures or both" (Doherty and Hicks 1977). Also, it should not be assumed that the costs of care for an individual in any program is equal to the individual's total life-support costs.

## Protective Services

As has been noted earlier, getting a person into the appropriate level of care, at the right time, is one critical factor for the successful delivery of services. Mentally and physically infirm older people may, however, on occasion need help from an objective, unrelated party to sort out the options for care. This is particularly important if, as is sometimes the case, an inappropriate decision may actually increase the individual's frailty or risk.

It is estimated that mentally and physically infirm older persons needing protective services number in excess of two million, and that an equal number are totally dependent on the support of relatives, friends, or social service agencies (Regan and Sprenger 1977). Beyond the questions of the right and ability to select appropriate services is the additional complicated issue of the protection and appropriate use of an older person's real assets. Newspapers regularly report "con games" designed to take advantage of lonely older people seeking to be helpful or to gain friends, but the ongoing abuse of the resources of the frail older person is undoubtedly more pervasive than the isolated confidence scheme. Older people have been frightened into poor investment decisions, insurance purchases, or excessive expenditures for services because of their inability to defend adequately their own interests or understand the reality of the money market.

Social agencies have typically defended the rights of the frail older person and urged their protection. However, many of the issues of protective services require the legal protection and effective functioning of a legal service organization that can provide consistent, available resources. Such a legal service organization should be integrated into the full network of services in the continuum and treated as part of the entitlement services every older person has a right to expect from society.

Protective services have been defined as:

> . . . an interdisciplinary program of assistance to persons with mental and physical disabilities, who can no longer take care of their basic needs, and who require community support. The underlying factor is the potential for legal intervention in the beneficiary's life. Such intervention, in principle, is invoked for a person who is not capable of making decisions in personal or business matters and is dangerous or is in danger. Some have interpreted this principle to mean that legal intervention may be invoked when a person refuses services deemed by others to be necessary to the safety of the beneficiary or the public. (Regan and Sprenger 1977)

Legal intervention may take any of the following forms outlined by Regan and Sprenger (1977): civil commitment to an institution; guardianship, which transfers control over personal decision making; guardianship (conservatorship) of the individual's property, which transfers control over property and financial affairs; protective service laws authorizing temporary intervention and protective placements. When these services are accepted voluntarily there may be no need for legal intervention because the services are considered to be supportive instead of protective. When the individual does require protective services, however, attention must be given to sustaining the individual's personal sense of dignity even though some basic rights are reduced. Care must be taken to remove only those rights that are essential for the individual's and society's protection. Where the supportive services can be provided by a caretaker, this should be encouraged; when the older person demonstrates restored ability to conduct his own affairs, the legal protection should be withdrawn, thereby reinstating the individual's freedom and rights.

Other systems available to protect the rights of older persons include emergency intervention, power of attorney, a substitute payee, creation of a trust, and joint tenancy. Each option should be evaluated for its appropriateness to the problems identified.

It should be expected that the need for any level of protective services would be explored during the assessment part of admission into the system and that the prescription for services would be implemented by the case manager. Acknowledging that there is need for a public guardian for those individuals without funds to purchase services is another aspect of acceptance of the idea that the frail older person has an entitlement to a full range of protective services.

# Advocacy

It is important that chronically ill older people be represented by constructively critical advocates of their needs and rights. Advocacy can take the form of membership on a governing board of a service agency. While advocacy can be viewed as an inherent role of such governing boards, this form may not always be most representative of the needs of the clients. Members of a governing board often establish strong identification with the organization and its management problems, so an independent advocate organization also is needed to provide another option for the aggrieved individual or to argue on behalf of characteristics of the system or services that will ultimately benefit all users.

Advocacy for improvement or modification of services may be the accepted role for any of several organizations. These need not necessarily be identified as organizations of older people; inappropriate or insufficient service to the older chronically ill person should be the concern of all members of our society. One possible approach could be the establishment of a community advisory board, charged specifically with providing critical analysis of the programs and services and advising the governing board on issues facing the older person.

Another effective advocate is an ombudsman, a respected community resource who attempts to resolve issues through open discussion, investigation of issues, and conciliatory efforts. The ombudsman is especially valuable because, in contrast to an advisory committee that will argue on behalf of clients, he or she represents a specific resource to older persons who are not adept at maneuvering their way through the bureaucratic mazes that stand between them and specific services. The ombudsman can be seen as an impartial, personal advocate ready to help older people gain access to their entitlements. Since chronically ill older people may, by nature of their illness, be dependent and incapable of personal advocacy, an effective long-term care system must include both an advocacy program and protective services.

The major responsibility for advocacy on the national level has been assigned to the Administration on Aging, and is known as the Advocacy Assistance Program. This program represents: "The convergence of two programs begun in 1975, one dealing with the development of nursing home ombudsman activities and the other with legal services support functions" (Sicker 1979). An earlier HEW Nursing Home Ombudsman Demonstration Program led to a recommendation that an ongoing ombudsman program be established in every state, with preference given for its location in the state unit on aging. The Administration on Aging Nursing Home

Ombudsman Program was formally established in 1975 to serve as the focal point for the promotion and development of nursing home ombudsman activities in each state.

Administration on Aging legal services activities also were initiated in 1975, and were intended to improve the general well-being of older people. While the ombudsman program was focused exclusively on the needs of nursing home patients, the legal services program gave little attention to the needs of the institutionalized aged. As a result, in 1978, the two programs were restructured into the Older Americans Advocacy Assistance Program, "with the mission of assisting the aging network in securing new rights, benefits, and entitlements for older persons, with particular emphasis on the most vulnerable elderly both in and out of long-term care institutions" (Sicker 1979).

The functions of the advocacy assistance program have been grouped into three broad areas. These are: (1) *personal advocacy,* developing programs to assist individuals living in nursing homes or with issues such as supplementary security income, food stamps, guardianship, pensions, consumer affairs, and housing; (2) *issues advocacy,* responding to the concerns affecting large numbers of older people, living at home or in an institution. Support services are to be provided for dealing with policy, regulation, and legislation; (3) *training and technical assistance,* offering help with the design and coordination of training programs that enable those who serve the aging to pursue personal and issues advocacy (Sicker 1979).

Advocacy at the national level has also been the responsibility of the leadership of national organizations representing the elderly. These groups have been organized as the Ad Hoc Leadership Council of Aging organizations and have advocated a national policy on aging as well as support for varied programs serving the elderly (Crowley and Cloud 1979).

The effective advocate role need not always be perceived as existing outside of the service organization. In fact, it should be the responsibility of every professionally trained person employed in long-term care to serve as an advocate on behalf of older people receiving appropriate care and entitlements from the long-term care system. Long-term care administrators, because they represent professional leadership in long-term care, have the added responsibility of setting standards and providing assertive role models for others in the field. The leadership demonstrated by administrators will in a large measure set the expectations for performance from all of the long-term care employees, and will go a long way toward assuring fair and appropriate services for all who require long-term care.

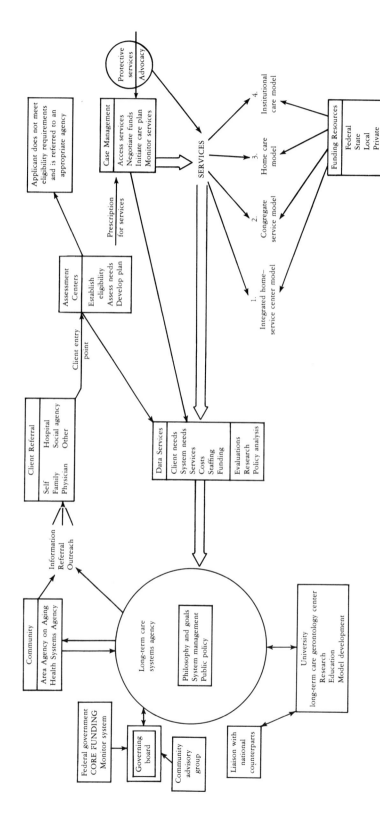

Fig. 6. The Long-Term Care System: Its Components and Context

## Summary

Figure 6 provides a summary of the long-term care system, illustrating the relationship between the major units in the core system, the services, funding, central adminstration, and relationship to the community. Major portions of this system are already operational for limited populations in select communities throughout the country. With increased support from the federal government, comparable systems can be established in metropolitan areas. Critical to this development is the ability of local communities to package their systems in a way that is compatible with their own resources, while assuring that the major characteristics of the system are included.

# Chapter

# 6

# The Management of Human Resources

*The secret of the care of the patient is in caring for the patient.*

FRANCIS W. PEABODY, M.D.

*The director of a relatively very good but large general hospital once remarked that his institution had been provided with almost lavish facilities and with an amazingly generous supply of professionally trained persons of all kinds. The problem, said he, was how the hospital could learn to use its human resources as well as it had learned to use diagnostic procedures and treatment facilities, including complex machines.*

ESTHER LUCILE BROWN, PH.D.

If the long-term care program is to be successful it will be because the employees of the organization make it so. The program recommended here is composed of a loose federation of autonomous groups, each of which would have primary responsibility to its own organization and a secondary allegiance to the coordinating structure of the long-term care system. The long-term care organization's control over public funds does not insure commitment to it from each of the federation's partners. Staff members need to feel that the sense of accomplishment they achieve is enhanced by participating in a long-term care organization offering a quality of service better than any individual organization could produce alone. Staff members can best develop a sense of belonging to the larger long-term care system through a program that provides opportunities for growth and advancement superior to the offerings of any single organization in the system. Such a program also leads to greater identification of staff with long-term care.

Managing the personnel of a participating organization or that of the coordinating long-term care organization involves similar responsibilities, differing only according to the labor intensity of each program. Obviously institutional care programs are the most labor-intensive. For example, the number of employees of nursing homes increased 850 percent between 1960 and 1978. Of the more than 951,000 people who work in nursing homes, 45 percent are aides and orderlies, 7 percent are professional nurses, and 9 percent are licensed practical nurses. Housekeeping and laundry workers' wages have increased 7 percent, dietitians accounted for 1 percent, and clerical workers for 3 percent (Schock 1981). Employee absenteeism can create a major budget crisis when last minute arrangements have to be made for temporary employees. This problem not only can force the institution out of compliance with licensing rules for staffing, but can also generally undermine the ability of the institution to carry out its service responsibilities. Frequent turnover of personnel creates the additional burden of replacing staff, with attendant costs of recruiting and training, and disrupts the continuity of the caring relationship between staff members and residents.

Employees in long-term care, whether in the coordinating or direct service function, can be drawn together by their identification with the people and purposes of the organization. Acknowledging this in no way reduces the importance of salaries, fringe benefits, and working conditions; however, as salaries and fringe benefits become standardized through minimum wages or agreed upon community standards, job satisfaction and opportunities for creative participation and advancement become increasingly important. Where there are significant differences between salaries for workers in acute and long-term care, employees may be attracted to the acute care settings in spite of their desire to work in long-term care.

## Attitudes Toward Aging and Illness

Development of staff programs in long-term care should be approached at two different levels: encouraging people to want to work with the frail elderly and keeping employees motivated to meet the goals of the employing organization. A key factor in attracting suitable employees to the field of long-term care is discovering attitudes toward aging and illness. Prospective employees may have attitudes about working with the aged that reflect the negative values our society attaches to aging and the aged. Available research supports the contention that professionals in health related fields hold negative attitudes toward the elderly. Surely the attitudes of health care professionals will affect the type and quality of care given the aged (Cyrus-Lutz and Gaitz 1972). In a study of medical students' attitudes, prejudice against the aged was noted to be even stronger than prejudice against color (Spence and Veigenbaum 1968).

In "The Reluctant Therapist," Kastenbaum (1963) examined "some of the unexamined attitudes which psychotherapists frequently hold in respect to the aged." The author suggests that these attitudes tend to block efforts at psychotherapy and derive from the clinician's failure to disentangle himself or herself from biases and misunderstandings prevalent in our society. These include the relatively low status assigned the elderly, the inability of clinicians to disassociate themselves from their own aging process, and the assumption that such efforts are of little benefit to those who do not have long to live.

Cyrus-Lutz and Gaitz (1972) discovered that psychiatric students they queried felt that the talents of a brilliant therapist would be wasted on the aged. This prejudice was equally strong among freshman and senior medical students. A typical attitude expressed was that the older person would not live long enough to pay back the therapist's investment.

In a later study, Gruber (1977) concluded that: "The attitudes of the doctor and the doctor-in-training toward the old usually are considered to be products of these primary influences: (1) the pervasive societal negativity toward aged people in general, and (2) the medical setting, acquired by virtue of the physician's unique training and experience as well as the emulation of his role models." In that same study, physicians responded to a questionnaire about geriatric medicine by saying, "It is too depressing, patients are difficult, and there is little medicine and doctors can do for these patients." Other physicians responded that because the patient will not get well again, the physician feels he has failed. Some said they had inadequate knowledge of chronic illness.

According to Wilson and Hafferty (1980):

> Medical professionals have often viewed the elderly through a cultural lens that focuses on deterioration, dependency, rigidity, and resistance to treatment. The treatment of chronic conditions is often viewed as less than appealing by a specialist-oriented medical profession. Such attitudes can influence the type of care provided to the elderly and so alter

expectations about the elderly that treatable illnesses are misdiagnosed. If the growing health needs of the elderly are to be effectively met, attitudes toward the elderly must be improved.

An experiment in medical education that resulted in more favorable attitudes toward the elderly was reported by Wilson and Hafferty (1980) as part of a seminar on aging and health offered to first year medical students. "Factors considered important in changing attitudes toward the elderly were factual information, personal contact with sick and well elderly, personal contact with role models for clinical geriatrics, and student case presentation of elderly patients."

Studies of nurses' attitudes revealed some of the same negative feelings. Nursing personnel prefer younger persons and younger patients. There was also some correlation between the nurse's age and the preferred age of patients. Salary increase or shift preference did not significantly increase the willingness of a nurse to work with elderly patients. Campbell (1971) also found that licensed practical nurses and nursing aides were more willing to work with the elderly than were registered nurses. There may be a correlation between the lower level of education and willingness to work with the elderly; or, conversely, nursing students may feel that advanced education is wasted on the elderly.

In a review of the literature, Robb (1979) found that nursing students and registered nurses expressed more unwillingness or reluctance to work with elderly clients in general hospitals and nursing homes than with clients in other age groups. Robb also found that students who completed a structured experience with healthy elderly people expressed a strong interest in working with the elderly. Robb also said that, because the elderly are undervalued by society, those nurses who express interest in working with the elderly are also undervalued. This transfer of values may extend to all who work with the elderly.

Geiger (1978) examined the way social work, law, and medical students view the elderly and found that the students lacked basic knowledge about the aged. None of the students gave first preference to working with the elderly in their future careers. She concluded that, "students in the helping professions are disinclined to work with the elderly despite their apparent belief that there is a large percentage of old people with important problems." She also noted that none of the three relevant professional schools required a course specifically on aging.

Solomon and Vickers (1979) found that stereotyping older people could result in the provision of unnecessary services. They also observed that close contact in a positive context resulted in a reduction of stereotyping and more individualization, whereas close contact in a negative context reinforced prejudicial stereotyping. Student nurses who resented their assignment to care for older patients increased their stereotyping of older people despite the availability of corrective information. Finally, Solomon and Vickers (1979) conclude that: "It is the geriatric treatment milieu, rather than the knowledge, experience, and skill of the staff, which affects attitudes, and little change appears to have taken place in attitudes toward the aging over the past twenty-five to thirty years."

The studies cited illustrate that many efforts have been made to better understand how to attract professionals to the care of the elderly. It is clear that health professionals generally are reluctant to work with the frail elderly. Prejudicial stereotypes may also impair the quality of services provided. It is not clear what educational experiences might either change the stereotypes or make working with the elderly more attractive. Modifying the working environment, providing opportunities to work with the well elderly, and especially communicating a sense of value to the professional's contribution, may be the most effective ways to attract people to work in long-term care. In a sense, then, the newness of the long-term care system, the value of the assessment center and case management, as well as the care plan representing the treatment of choice by a multidisciplinary group of care providers, may add a sense of qualitative difference or newness and increase the field's attractiveness to health professionals. It has also been suggested (Schock 1981) that affiliation between a university and long-term care programs might enhance the value of working in long-term care if the university uses it for research, education, and program development. This is in keeping with the intended benefits of affiliation with the new long-term care gerontology centers.

## Multidisciplinary Teams

Implementation of a long-term care program will depend upon the successful integration of the strengths and resources of a multidisciplinary team of care providers. The multidisciplinary team is composed of the varied professional disciplines involved in the provision of long-term care services. There may be hierarchical differences within the team, defined by position or title, education, or length of employment, and there is no point in artificially denying these differences. However, each team member should be recognized for his or her legitimate role on the team. Roles need not be static and positions in the team structure can change as members grow in their personal strength and professional skills.

The team concept is important because providing care for those who are chronically ill usually involves multiple disciplines relating to the individual's medical, social, environmental, and economic problems. Leadership of this unique team in long-term care is often assigned to the case manager, but the case manager may in fact be a family member or the person for whom the entire system is designed to provide care.

## Staff Development

These ideas are basic to differentiating between the approaches of in-service education and staff development. In-service education provides education and training to the employees; staff development, in contrast, attempts to develop an environment in which staff can grow and mature, can make significant contributions to the organization, and can gain a sense of accomplishment through their participation.

For example, the loose federation of autonomous care providers who make up the long-term care continuum provides options for employment at different levels of administration and direct service. Within this continuum of services to the elderly there are opportunities for a range of employment experiences that can support job enrichment and career ladders for upward mobility. Positions defined as entry level can have promotional opportunities throughout the continuum instead of within a single agency. Job rotation through several agencies in the continuum will add to the variety of employment opportunities, open up new challenges, and contribute to the sense of a common goal through the exchange of employees. It is possible that a plan of this scope would offset some of the negative attitudes toward working with the elderly and provide an incentive for employment.

### Hiring

To encourage this process, applicants should be interviewed by a personnel committee made up of representatives of a variety of care components, including an institution, a senior center, and a home care program. This group would be able to discuss the range of services available and contribute a sense of the total program of long-term care.

Additionally, representatives of the group of frail elderly using the services can make an important contribution in staff selection, especially by urging that services be planned with the recipients of the service involved from the outset. This reinforces the point made earlier that older people and their families should be involved in the prescription for services and may modify or reject the recommendations of the assessment team. Placing an older person on the team selecting new employees should communicate to the applicant that these people are valued participants in the process as well as recipients of the services offered. Because the long-term care program will be providing services to older people with varying levels of chronic illness, it should be relatively easy to find capable older persons to represent the service agencies. This representation would be more difficult to obtain for those organizations serving only the most severely chronically ill.

It is important to begin any employment interview with a statement of purpose of the organization or long-term care system. This simple statement should be clearly understood by each employee and, more importantly, inspire each employee to accept it as the statement of a personal mission in the organization. Leaders of the organization can initiate the process of identifying the right kind of employee by demonstrating how the organization is true to its standards and how these standards help older people function more effectively. The bond that unifies loosely federated agencies or different shifts in an institution is the bond of service that brings the greatest reward to the employee. For example, every employee should be convinced that his or her presence on the job each day is of great value to the organization, especially to the older people served.

*Incentives*

Leaders of organizations in long-term care know from experience that their own behavior toward every employee serves as a model for expectations of the employee's behavior in relating to an older person in the program. A new staff orientation program should include observation of the assessment process, the role of the case manager, and of selected services other than the one in which the person will be employed. The employee should be given a complete overview of the long-term care program. Specific content of the employee's job, personnel practices, and all other appropriate content should also be described.

In a study of the training of unlicensed long-term care personnel, Feldman, Burke, and Schwarzmann (1978) comment on the difficult problems of high staff turnover and its impact on the cost of long-term care. They cite lack of career mobility as a major reason for personnel leaving their jobs. The availability of a personnel market in the long-term care system that is significantly larger than any one of the participant organizations lends itself to a variety of explorations of career mobility within the system through job rotation. Scholarship programs to enable career growth might also encourage employees to remain in the field. For example, nursing attendants could be given financial support to attend classes in order to advance to practical or registered nursing.

An enlarged personnel pool also lends itself to a variety of social activities to give employees a chance to meet others in the system and to derive a sense of social recognition associated with employment. A bowling team, weekend picnic, or holiday party may all be part of a series of events that help bring staff together.

Opportunities should be taken to give recognition to outstanding personnel contributions, including, for example, cost saving procedures, best attendance records, and long tenure. It should go without saying that none of these is a substitute for a suitable salary, which is the minimum requirement of good personnel practice. Social activities and opportunities for recognition, like development of personnel practices, should involve the employees. Representatives of employee groups should participate with owners or managers in developing the total package of employment benefits.

*Education and Training*

Despite the resources that have been channeled into programs serving the aged and chronically ill, the needs of the population may not be adequately met. One reason is that the personnel available to established, innovative, and new programs are often untrained or ill-prepared. Achievement of program goals with personnel who are not properly oriented or who lack necessary knowledge and skills is made very difficult (Feldman, Burke, and Schwarzmann 1978). Continuing education has been a major resource for upgrading performance skills and communicating new information, but participation in classes does not guarantee learning (Mote 1976). Nor is learning enhanced if the class sessions are offered at the end of a busy day or sandwiched between other demands. People learn because they want to learn or need to learn. Students should be involved in setting the topics, schedules, and settings for classes.

While evaluation of continuing education has been limited in terms of changed behavior or improvement in the quality of care, responsibility to the recipients of the care demands that continuing efforts be made to improve the quality of services offered. Continuing education is an important resource that can be supported through cooperative arrangements with local colleges or universities. One example of this is the coordinated training offered by the University of Arizona program in Long-Term Care Administration and the Pima County Community Services System (Monahan and Koff 1979). The university program is responsible for most of the training provided to all employees in that local long-term care network, to older people, and to the community at large.

Hinkley (1978) defines staff development in long-term care as "an ongoing educational/training program that addresses itself to the learning needs of staff, residents, and families that are relevant to the provision of quality care." Some typical components of a staff development program include orientation, skill training, organization and team building skills, analysis of characteristics of the service population, and general procedures such as fire safety, patients' rights, and so on. It is important to involve staff in the organizational development, statement of the philosophy of the organization, and development of personnel practices in order to enhance each employee's understanding of how the total organization operates. A wide range of participation in policy development will ultimately result in products that reflect contributions from many devoted employees. Staff development provides opportunities for employees to participate in meaningful experiences in the administration of the organization, thereby increasing their understanding and skills. A successful outgrowth of this level of involvement could be expansion of the classical management team of department heads or administrators to include other employees who have demonstrated their abilities and are ready to move up the ladder of responsibilities.

One of the advantages of the long-term care organization is that it provides varied work opportunities, more qualitative educational experiences, an assortment of social activities, and participation in staff development that can enhance each employee's growth and contribution to the organization. These opportunities may offset some of the negative attitudes about working in the field of long-term care and help to attract better qualified persons to work with the frail elderly.

## A Caring Philosophy

According to Solomon (1981): "Older people in long-term care suffer from simultaneous physical, emotional and social assaults. Despite these assaults, with the help of family and caretakers, they continue, as they always have, to battle for survival. New adaptive tasks are posed for them at every turn—a move to a new neighborhood, a move to a child's home, survival on a small fixed income, creating a new life-style commensurate with increasing physical disability."

In the delivery of long-term care services, the philosophy that binds together the goals and services is the commitment to caring. This caring is especially important in long-term care because of the increasing numbers in need, the frailty of each participant, and general public apathy regarding care of the frail elderly. Every person involved in long-term care must be prepared not only to contribute the highest level of skills and expertise, but also to communicate a caring attitude. The frail older person, having experienced losses through chronic illness and withdrawal from the mainstream of society, needs to sense caring concern.

Philabert (1976) describes caring for the frail elderly as a threefold task that includes: helping to restore the person's health; alleviating the person's suffering and decreasing incapacities; accompanying the person through the illness even when there is no certainty or hope at all of a cure and when suffering and/or handicaps cannot be alleviated to any extent.

Philabert's message is clearly that of a consistent caring even when hope of cure is absent. And when cure is absent, hope is not abandoned. Caring can also be expressed by enabling the older person to exercise choices among the options available. The absence of choice confirms one's disadvantaged status. Caring can be expressed by avoiding professional judgments about what is best for the person with chronic illness, and instead providing situations where older people can decide what is in their own best interest (Solomon 1981).

To care is to be anxious, to be concerned, to be inclined or disposed to like or to love. Fromm describes love "as the deepest need of man to overcome his separateness, to leave the prison of his aloneness" (1956). The basic elements of love in Fromm's thesis are care, responsibility, respect, and knowledge. In long-term care, responsibility could easily deteriorate into domination and possessiveness—the antithesis of love—were it not for showing respect and the ability to be aware of each person's uniqueness and individuality. These ideas are comparable to those of Mayeroff (1971) in his essay "On Caring": "To care for another person, in the most significant sense, is to help him grow and actualize himself." Mayeroff identifies five major ingredients of caring which are especially germane to long-term care. These include:

1. *Knowing.* To care for someone we must know many things about the person, what is conducive to growth, what are the strengths and limitations, what are the needs and aspirations. We need to know who the person is we are caring for as well as know ourselves, our powers and limitations.
2. *Reappraisal.* While we learn and mature from earlier experiences, it is essential that we not assume that any person will be like any other person. Each circumstance requires a reappraisal so that the individual in need is not presumed to have any stereotyped characteristics.

3. *Patience.* This reflects an attitude of hope and the willingness to maintain the caring even if the older person is not capable of mustering quick responses. Patience also is demonstrated in the belief in the ability of the person to grow.
4. *Honesty.* We must not merely tell the truth but must permit ourselves to understand and to react to circumstances.
5. *Trust.* We must achieve the ability to let go, to trust by not dominating. Trust also implies confidence in one's own capacity to care.

In addition, caring assumes continuity, and it is impossible to have a caring relationship when care providers are frequently replaced. The unmeasured cost of staff turnover is the disruption of caring relationships and the impact of this disruption on the morale and self-perceptions of those served by long-term care.

Brown (1961) points out that "care designed to meet psychosocial needs which rests primarily upon dynamic interpersonal relationships between staff and patients is exceedingly hard to achieve." Hence, she argues, it becomes exceedingly important to seek other ways of supplementing what is achieved through relationships. One of the most obvious of these is the planned use of the physical and social environments with which the older person comes in contact. Appropriate environments that contribute to a person's comfort express caring. It is important, for example, to provide calendars and clocks in institutional environments, lighting should be effective, printed materials should be readable, temperature controls should be accessible to the residents and users, and environments should be barrier-free.

Whenever we give up hope, display negative expectations because of a person's age, or treat people as if they and their illnesses are part of a homogenous group, we tend to dehumanize them. Especially in responding to the needs of those who have chronic illness, when little can be done to offset the ravages of the illness, active caring is the most comforting contribution that can be made.

The ability of staff to contribute to a caring relationship is probably enhanced by the way in which staff members feel the caring concern of their employers. It is inconsistent for staff to be treated in a demeaning way by their employers while being expected to act in a caring way with their older patients. Conversely, the ability to manage human resources to provide caring support for the older people should be demonstrated by similar treatment of employees.

Brown (1961) distinguishes five aspects of human personality that need nurturing by employers. These are:

1. *Social approval.* People gain social approval by working, by performing socially acceptable work, and by being valued for

their work. Unfortunately people who work with the frail elderly do not generally receive social approval for what they do. Because the frail older person does not have high status in our society, the work performed in caring for this group is also given low status. But work is important for social approval and the internal employer approval has to be evident to overcome possible negative aspects of the job and support the employee.

2. *Sense of accomplishment.* Work provides an important way of feeling a sense of accomplishment or value from the work effort. However, when much of the worktime is devoted to the frail elderly or those who will not necessarily enjoy an improvement in health or competence because of the work effort, the sense of accomplishment may be minimized. It is important to note for the employee that when cure is not possible caring remains of great importance and is appreciated. The sense of accomplishment can come for the quality of caring.

3. *Sense of the importance of the job.* A sense of job importance is very much related to social approval and accomplishment. All persons participating as part of the health care team need to be recognized for their importance.

4. *Security.* Security often refers to continuity of work, maintenance of salary and benefits, and the continuity of work related benefits, such as social contacts, sense of accomplishment, and social approval.

5. *Support in anxiety-inducing situations.* Working with older, frail persons unquestionably engenders personal feelings of dependency, incompetence, and anxiety about death. Many health care providers have not been adequately prepared to encounter these anxiety-inducing situations and need the ongoing understanding and support of their employers to assist them to function under these adverse circumstances.

## Summary

While we can't be assured of the most qualified, devoted staff at all times, or of the absence of staff turnover, we can take constructive measures to enable employees to achieve maximum levels of productivity. Essential to achieving this goal is an approach described as staff development, in which staff members are recognized for their contributions, are encouraged to participate in the policies and management of the organization, and are given the tools and support structure essential to well-managed human service programs.

It is obvious that attitudes about working with the frail elderly will influence a person's decision to work in long-term care, and will determine the effectiveness of the employee. Because of its multiple levels of entry for employees, and its varied opportunities in institutional care, home care, and management, the long-term care system provides options for job rotation and job variations that can be stimulating and enriching to the employee. The value of assessment, case management, multidisciplinary team planning, and multiple levels of services may increase the attractiveness of employment, possibly offsetting some of the negative aspects of working with the elderly. Placing older persons on employee interviewing committees should communicate to the applicant that the older person is considered as having worth and is a participant in the process as well as a recipient of the services offered.

In long-term care, where cures or hope for cures for chronic illness may be impossible, there should still be caring concern. Every participant in long-term care should appreciate the importance of a caring approach. Especially for older persons who suffer from the simultaneous physical, emotional, and social assaults, consistent solace can be provided by active, continuous caring.

# Chapter

# 7

# A System
# Responsive
# to
# Need

*Above all, do no harm.*

## The Search for Dignified, Efficient Care

While caring should be part of all health and social services, it is an essential ingredient of long-term care because where cure is not likely, caring becomes even more important. But caring is not the only quality by which long-term care should be assessed. Services should be available when they are needed, and should be administered so that the available resources are most efficiently and effectively used.

Tibbitts (1977) elaborates on the theme of the purpose of care of the chronically ill older person as

> . . . the provision of health facilities, programs, and services which enable aging and older people to enjoy the highest quality of life compatible with their physical and mental potentials in the light of available knowledge and resources and without regard for economic status. [This] . . . includes the elements necessary to prevent or postpone physical and mental breakdown, to support maintenance and restoration of health and preservation of independence when chronic illness and disabilities appear, and to afford whatever services may be required when older people are no longer able to cope with biomedical

and psychological changes and insults and with socioeconomic deprivations.

Inherent in this statement are related themes that deal with the just distribution of resources, the appropriateness of the services, clients' expectations of the services, the expertness of the services, and the efficiency of their delivery. This wide range of services, coordinated in a long-term care system and available to all who may require them, may not be possible to implement immediately, but is still a desirable goal.

While not all older people need long-term care services, society should have the capacity to respond to the changing needs and expectations of older people and the chronically ill in the same way libraries, parks, public health services, and educational institutions respond to the needs of the general populace today. Kahn and Kamerman (1976) describe this concept of "social utility" as representing the expectations of average citizens in our society in the normal conduct of their lives. Such expectations should be expanded to respond to the presence of large numbers of older people among us, and their special needs should be accepted as normal and not necessarily associated with illness or incapacity. The "constellation of community services" (Tibbitts 1977) developed as social utilities should include educational, social, and recreational opportunities for everyone to enjoy the best quality of life possible, as well as the preventive and restorative services to retain maximum health and vigor. It should be obvious that only through supportive public policies can the old, and especially the very old, have access to the full constellation of community resources considered to be essential to maintain a life of dignity.

# Rationing

Even though most people prefer aging to its only alternative, the elderly, as a group, is often regarded as an unwelcome component in our society. The elderly are often the poor of our communities, are seldom afforded the respected elder role, and are unfavorably measured by standards that idealize prolonged youthfulness. When a question is raised of allocating limited resources to children or the elderly, it is often argued that investment in children will be productive for a lifetime, that in older people only briefly. Within this framework, the older person does not fare well. As a result, society at large loses, because what is required is balance and just distribution for all groups and ages.

Even in the context of a more equitable distribution of resources, however, there appears to be what Mechanic (1978) calls a requirement for "rationing" care services: "I value a system of medical care distribution that results in the highest level of effective outcome, reduced disability, and enhanced comfort possible within a given range of available resources." When a decision must be made about distribution of service resources, how are the preferences of society to be determined and how can the merits of relative decisions and their impact on society be evaluated? "In reality, the needs of one social group or another are communicated by the ability of that group, or that of its advocates, to arouse an emotional response in those holding the powers of decision" (Mechanic 1978). The high cost factors associated with long-term care for increasing numbers of older people have been heavily emphasized in presentations of their needs. For example, the increasingly high costs of institutional care for a rapidly growing segment of the elderly have resulted in greater need for rationing resources, setting the stage for exploration of alternate resources to maintain older people in better health so they can remain at home and be less likely to need institutional care. It may be that an approach to the financing of institutional care that has ignored the possible need for rationing has benefited society by having created the need to develop and support a constellation of services.

Although overt rationing of services might not have worked well as a tool to restrict or equitably distribute services, another form of rationing may have emerged. It deals with the extent to which society is committed to caring for the chronically ill and is, in essence, a rationing of quality rather than quantity. For example, while health care providers do not deny their services to the chronically ill, they have for the most part not viewed serving the chronically ill as being of great importance, and have not valued expertise in caring for the chronically ill. The absence of professionals committed to the care of the chronically ill may, in fact, be evidence of a subtle rationing of interests, commitments, and resources to this segment of our population. Such rationing is alarming because it contradicts the assumption that enough public money and enough staff are all that are required for more responsible care. That same assumption also undermines the role of advocacy groups acting on behalf of the elderly to claim for them an appropriate share of available resources. If advocates' voices are stilled, the chronically ill elderly may not receive necessary services, even though large sums of money are expended.

An additional deterrent to the older person's receiving adequate health care is the barrier created by regulations governing coinsurance and deductibles. According to Mechanic (1978), "such cost-sharing features—very much like the direct fee—have greater inhibitory effects on the poor than on the more affluent and continue existing inequities in distribution." Deductibles and coinsurance are intended to help the consumer distinguish between basic and discretionary components of health care and thereby judge carefully before using the discretionary aspects. It is inappropriate, however, to expect the chronically ill person to make this distinction, or to assume that postponing or reducing the ready availability of care to the chronically ill person is a reasonable means of controlling health costs. Primary health care services for the chronically ill should be provided as an entitlement since eligibility requirements or other barriers to receiving required services may, in fact, result in unnecessary deterioration of health and eventually higher expenses.

Rationing may also be effected through allocative and regulatory decisions that deal with manpower and facility allocation, inclusion or exclusion of benefits, and social regulations of health care:

> Rationing can never be just in the sense that it promises each patient the same services or equal units of service . . . (nor can) rationing . . . promise that all patients with comparable problems will be treated alike. . . . Services have to be provided on an individual basis, responsive to the uniqueness of each individual and each circumstance. . . . In this context, justice refers not to any specific quantity or type of service but to the establishment of a rationing process that is as explicit as possible, and yet where the rules for rationing are based on sound clinical judgment, rather than on arbitrary social categorizations. (Mechanic, 1978)

Rationing is a crucial factor in the search for dignified, personal, efficient care for those who are chronically ill. Similarly, the search for quality services is influenced by a plethora of interwoven dynamics that make it difficult to develop and evaluate them. It is important to understand some of the major forces influencing the quality of services and it is essential to appreciate the dynamics of these relationships for developing, administering, or evaluating long-term care services. Figure 7 identifies some of these variables.

## Evaluating Quality

Brook (1977) has pointed out that evaluating quality is complicated, with no easy approaches or solutions; it has not contributed much to improving health care and it has become a big

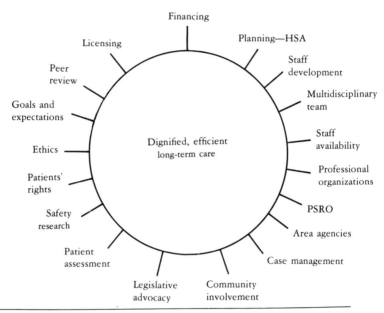

Fig. 7.  Variables Influencing the Shape and Responsiveness of Long-Term Care

business. With these thoughts in mind, it is probably most useful to discuss only those characteristics of the current vogue for evaluation that influence the emerging long-term care system. Essentially what is described here is an organizational approach committed to assuring quality services, rather than a process approach that would examine the effectiveness of services or an outcome approach that would focus on the state of health of those in the system. Evaluations may also be viewed as taking place concurrently with the delivery of services or retrospectively by looking at both outcome and process criteria measurements to permit evaluation of a pattern of care. Approaches for evaluating care can be found in Miller and Knapp (1979), Ainsworth (1972), Jones, Denson, and McNitt (1978), Professional Standards Review Organization (PSRO) literature, and many journal articles. Many of these approaches deal with institutional care, nursing services, or medical care. Other approaches may examine cost benefits of alternative services or methodologies in long-term care.

While each of these assesses some of the major portions of long-term care, there is as yet no systematic way of evaluating the full scope of the program. This is in no small way related to the problems of defining long-term care, its goals, and the components of a coordinated system. Criteria of quality must be established that can be understood and applied by each of the contributors to the total system. Goal statements are needed for the entire system and its administration, as well as for the care provided to each participant.

## *Ethics*

"Ethics deals with classification of things and events on the basis of the values attached to them. It is supposed to say whether this is good or bad" (Cottress 1977). However, because long-term care involves many people from a variety of backgrounds, as well as many different organizations, it is difficult to construct a single, simple ethical statement. The comprehensive long-term care organization must design its own code of ethics, capable of representing a common base of expected behavior consistently throughout all its components:

> The job of an administrator is to organize and allocate resources to accomplish an objective. In the case of long-term care administration, these resources are made up, to a great degree, by other professional individuals through whom care and services are provided. Thus, there must be assurance that their actions are consistent with the value system of the administrative profession. In order to do that, administrators must know, understand, and publicly affirm their values and beliefs. (Kuperberg 1978)

Many long term care administrators, however, are neither specially trained in long-term care nor affiliated with an association of long-term care administrators that has an identified code of ethics. There is no forum where a statement of long-term care administrators' ethics can be tested. Additionally, many of the employees in long-term care have not come through an academic discipline or educational program that has its own implicit or explicit code of ethics. It is, therefore, especially important that a normative set of ethics for long-term care be established to which all who work in the field can subscribe.

It is insufficient to say that each participant in the long-term care program can rely on his or her own ethical standards, given the disparity of backgrounds and changing values in our society. It is important to arrive at a statement of ethics that can unite all participants in a common approach to working with the chronically ill older person, working with public trust and public funds, and cooperating with a large group of employees to carry out the mission of the organization.

Medical ethics can be used to illustrate the problems health care practitioners face when trying to reconcile societal values with their own professional practice in long-term care. Medical views on aging reflect the broad spectrum of community values: "These are, on the one hand, the philosophy that the elderly have less social and moral value than other individuals, and, on the other hand, the view that they have greater value than other persons. Probably most health professionals fall between these extremes; however, it is important to recognize that both philosophies affect clinical decisions and for that reason it is important to recognize current expressions of these two positions" (Gadow 1980). Practitioners need some moral guidelines to respond to individual caring situations. Gadow advocates beneficence and autonomy as guiding principles. Beneficence requires "doing good," or taking action for clients to prevent harm to them, benefit them, or permit harm only when the harm is unavoidable and when it is significantly outweighed by the benefit. (See also the discussion of beneficence as it applies to research at the end of this chapter.) The principle of autonomy requires respect for the freedom of self-determination of those affected directly by a decision of a provider of care.

## Patients' Rights

The issue of patients' rights is intimately tied to that of ethics. Long-term care administrators must identify their ethical foundation and values in order to set guidelines for their administrative behavior. How they discharge an employee, handle a client's transfer of residence, protect cherished possessions, or respond to an elderly person who appears to be in need of a guardian are the kinds of issues that must be handled from an ethical perspective. It is easy for administrators to respond to dependent older people by assuming greater responsibility than is appropriate.

A patient's bill of rights is the counterpart of a code of ethics in that it is a reminder that the older person expects the administrator to behave in an ethical manner. The administrator in turn is responsible for communicating these ethical standards, expressed in the patients' bill of rights, to all other employees, and for assuring that employees understand the issues and incorporate the expected performance into their job responsibilities.

While the idea of a patients' bill of rights was first raised for skilled and intermediate care facilities because they served the most dependent older people, it is an idea that should be implemented at all levels of long-term care. If a statement of rights is to be more than a show of good intentions, it is vital that some means of enforcement be accessible to patients. According to Wilson (1978), the elderly person ". . . whose rights have been aggrieved is prevented from bringing suit by his isolation from the community, including lawyers; his lack of physical energy and psychic combativeness; the problems of proof where staff will unite against aged and drugged complainants; the law of damages which places small value on injury to those whose actuarial life expectancies are zero; and his probable lack of money to pay for legal representation." Older people in such a situation have been failed by the system upon which they depend. For this reason, a local, independent ombudsman who will jolt the local public protective and advocacy systems on behalf of the frail older person is an important part of the protection of rights in long-term care.

## Area Agency on Aging

The presence of a strong area agency on aging can be an effective resource for establishing a close liaison between community service agencies, organizations of older people, and the long-term care network. Certainly, where there is an established tradition to plan cooperatively for new or improved community services, the community service agencies may be more responsive to the cooperative requirements of long-term care. It is this responsiveness to community needs that can be effective in avoiding unnecessary duplication of services, competitiveness among the service providers, and a redirection of energies and funds into the most productive components. Cooperative planning to assure the availability of essential services and the flexibility to modify services in response to individualized requirements is necessary, and is more likely to be found where there is a functioning area agency on aging.

In addition, the area agency on aging can facilitate consumer participation in planning, implementing, and monitoring the long-term care system to enable the most effective participation of the older person in the system. The area agency on aging can help select, train, and support the older person who possesses the tools to provide valuable contributions to long-term care.

## Health Systems Agency

The Health Systems Agency (HSA) is responsible for planning to meet the health service needs of the entire community: "The HSA must by law determine health status goals and health systems goals for its area and propose recommended long-run programs for the accomplishment of these goals. A document called the Health Systems Plan articulates these long-run community goals and programs and must be made available to the community" (Dittman and Peters 1978). HSA's have had the greatest impact on the development of new health care organizations, especially institutional facilities, in avoiding unnecessary services, and in community review of charges for health services.

Cooperation among health care providers and community

leaders encourages greater appreciation for all components of health care and establishes an environment in which long-term care can function most effectively.

## Professional Standards Review Organization

PSRO was established by the 1972 Amendments to the Social Security Act (PL 92-603), and is intended to "ensure that professional standards are maintained in the provision of health care that is federally financed and to ensure that federal funds are expended in the most economical and efficient manner possible" (PSRO 1978).

The functions of PSRO are carried out by reviewing admissions to health care facilities, certifying the necessity for continued treatment in the facility, conducting medical care reviews, and reviewing extended or costly treatment. PSRO's have begun to extend their review into some of the long-term care facility programs receiving Medicaid support, and in a more limited way have initiated some demonstration programs for ambulatory care.

PSRO's represent an approach to assuring quality care in health care programs, principally through medical care review and influence over physicians as the principal decision makers. The person using long-term care services, however, is generally someone with chronic illnesses, has multiple medical and social problems, and requires a multidisciplinary approach. Admission into any of the long-term care services is generally not purely for medical reasons, and review of need must be based on all pertinent factors (Altieri et al. 1977). As a result, lengths of stay in long-term care facilities cannot be determined on the basis of medical diagnosis alone. While medical care review can contribute to the overall quality of long-term care, it cannot be applied in the same way it is in the acute care setting. Establishing multidisciplinary assessment centers as points of entry into the long-term care system lends itself to preadmission (in the sense of admission into the system and not merely the institution) evaluation and review by a PSRO or similar organization. The multidisciplinary approach requires that the PSRO team be composed of those professionals generally represented in the long-term care assessment process (Snyder and Engelman 1977).

The HSA is intended to function cooperatively with the PSRO in improving quality, rationalizing resource allocation, and controlling expenditures in the health care system: "PSROs share with HSAs not only a fundamental purpose but also a local/regional structure; and thus the two types of organizations are well-suited to provide each other with advice and technical support in areas of mutual interest. Examples of key concerns shared by PSROs and HSAs are the appropriate supply and utilization of acute care and long-term care beds and the proper application of various health care services and technologies. (PSRO 1978)

## Peer Review

An alternate plan for incorporating the PSRO into the long-term care system would be to develop a multidisciplinary peer review of the process used by each of the disciplines represented. A committee to direct this effort should include consumer representatives in addition to representatives of the respective disciplines. This group should adopt standards for professional services, review subcommittee findings related to each profession, assess the quality of service and define unresolved problems, and report regularly to the management committee of the long-term care system (Deuschle et al. 1978).

The interaction of professional representatives on the peer review committee should complement multidisciplinary involvement in the overall management of the long-term care system. Those disciplines not usually represented on the peer review committee should be included to establish performance specifications for each of their disciplines.

## Professional Organizations

Whether groups of employees are referred to as professional organizations or trade associations does not influence their ability to have impact on the quality of services provided to older people. Their contribution is to assert standards of performance and find appropriate ways to measure compliance with those standards. These groups can also foster continuing participation in educational programs as a requirement for maintaining status in the organization. Beyond overseeing standards and compliance, these organizations can contribute to the stature of those involved in long-term care by their recognition of members' involvement as a valuable professional contribution. Peer acceptance and recognition support the value of the individual's work and thereby his or her worth to the peer group and community.

## Staff Availability

It is often difficult for staff who work with chronically ill people to gain a sense of worth from their work. A society that values individual productivity as highly as ours gives relatively low priority to work devoted to the chronically ill. The field of long-term care has had difficulty attracting workers and has reinforced its image of secondary status by offering salaries that are frequently less than those for comparable work with the acutely ill patient.

Staff interested in the chronically ill and qualified to work with them are essential to the development of quality programs. Educational institutions can contribute to the personnel pool if they recognize the significance of chronic illness in our society and incorporate appropriate classes and class content to prepare the practitioner. Competence in the field must include both technical skills and sensitive appreciation of the needs of those who suffer from long-standing disabling illnesses.

## Patient Assessment and Case Management

While both patient assessment and case management have been discussed earlier, it is important to refer to them again as we summarize some of the ways high standards and services can be built into long-term care programs. Quality care cannot be provided unless the needs of the older person are established in a thorough assessment. At the same time, if we cannot get older people to the needed services, and if appropriate follow-up is not provided, those people will not benefit from the assessment. Case management and assessment are the basic service processes essential to a program in long-term care.

## Financing

The ubiquitous problems of money are nowhere of greater concern than in the area of developing a quality long-term care program, but having enough money—however much that may be—is no assurance that it will be used to purchase the best services. Only if sufficient funds are accompanied by all the other related factors in program development can they be used to buy appropriate care. Money designated for only the most intensive level of care, resorted to when everything else has failed, is likely to be spent too late to be used most effectively. Money committed to research, training, and preventive sources, if used appropriately, is much more likely to be spent in support of the individual's independence and independent functioning.

# Research

Research can be an important component in the evolution of quality programs if it is related to improving the quality of services, seeking new services, and searching for answers to the causes and problems of chronic illnesses and disabilities. It seems appropriate to advocate that research programs in long-term care have close ties to the organized service system and be responsive to researchable issues raised through the provision of comprehensive services.

At the same time, the emphasis placed on research does not give license to abrogate the human rights of older people. Exploitation of human subjects cannot be justified even for the ultimate value of the successful research. Protection of human subjects is of great importance, especially when they may be frail older people unable to protect themselves adequately against the authority or power of the researchers. Just as older persons are less capable of putting off the persuasive requests of researchers, they are more prone to adverse reactions from exploitative behavior. Reich (1978) provides a framework for research that refers to three ethical principles applied to standards for research: beneficence, which affirms that we ought to produce good and prevent harm; just distribution, which requires a fair and equitable distribution of benefits and burdens; and respect, which protects and promotes the dignity and autonomy of individuals. Research with elderly subjects can be safely conducted only within these guidelines.

# Licensing and Regulation

Licensing and regulation processes affect the way long-term care services are provided because they control the supply of services, regulate costs and changes, assert standards, and monitor and control financial resources. Implemented together or separately these processes are not enough to support the development of quality services. According to Ruchlin (1977): "Although the long-term care sector is already subject to extensive regulation, these regulatory efforts have not brought about the desired levels of performance. The factors that have contributed to this failure are complex (inadequate financing, poor knowledge base). To some degree they are inherent in the traditional regulatory approach (bureaucratic apathy, political consideration). Moreover, some may not be amenable to change unless they are addressed directly as social problems rather than as problems unique to the long-term care sector (legal constraints, political considerations)."

Ruchlin further urges the association of the regulatory authority with local rate-setting and creation of a role for consumer groups in the overall regulatory process. In addition, rate-setting should be related to the "cost of providing the desired level of care in an economically efficient manner."

A long-term care system based on a service model uniquely related to the needs of the chronically ill is an alternative to the current regulatory mechanism, which has met with little success in assuring quality care for the chronically ill. This model examines social, residential, and health care needs in a constellation of essential services. It identifies the various contributors to a quality system, seeking to strengthen these resources and their relationship to the system to develop quality standards and competent delivery of services. Blending these services into a comprehensive system should be the focus for the coordination and administration of the entire effort. The Administration on Aging has suggested that these coordinating responsibilities be delegated to long-term care centers housed in major universities throughout the country (U.S. Dept. HEW Guidelines Older Americans Act 4E Program 1978). Efforts are currently under way to explore this possibility. These centers could emerge as the community focal point for the coordination of long term-care of chronically ill elderly people.

## Summary

The quality and quantity of services made available through the long-term care system are measured by various standards. The value we assign to the elderly and our commitments in public policy set the stage for the way we allocate our resources. We should also expect that providers of long-term care will be guided by the same ethical standards as all other health care professionals, adhering to a consistent ethic for long-term care. Inherent in this ethic should be a code of patients' rights to assure that older people be treated with dignity, be involved in the decisions affecting their lives, and be participants in the care system.

Some community agencies have special importance in determining the quality of long-term care, including the area agency on aging, the health systems agency, the professional standards review organization, and licensing agencies. Research and evaluation activities are an important part of long-term care, and should be guided by ethical considerations for the rights and privacy of older people.

# Chapter

# 8

# A Healthier
# Future:
# Many
# Happy
# Returns

*As we proceed in the next decade to develop a comprehensive national plan for care for the elderly, we urge that it include a range of options for patients and their families rather than depend on a pat formula. In a large, multiethnic, multiracial, geographically dispersed society such as the United States, local control and local imagination will be required to meet local programs creatively. The federal challenge is then to provide adequate inducements to ensure that care of the elderly is given sufficient priority in all areas of the country.*

ROBERT L. KANE
ROSALIE A. KANE

This book, so far, has offered an approach for a coordinated program of long-term care to respond to the needs of chronically ill older people. It is based on what one colleague refers to as the "worst-first idea" of having to respond to the needs of those persons who are chronically ill, and for whom the absence of a coordinated network of services has meant the absence of appropriate care. For the 10 percent to 15 percent of our population over the age of sixty-five who are in need of immediate services, there can be no option but to respond with the most sophisticated skills available to provide the most appropriate services. Public support for the plight of the chronically ill must be aroused. Reasonable funding to enable people to remain at their residence of choice for as long as possible must be assured and services must be developed and coordinated. The person in need of the services should not be coerced into accepting inappropriate care because adequate assessment of need cannot be made. Funds should be provided both for offering the appropriate level of service and assuring that the individual receives what is paid for—especially where public funds and responsibility are involved.

A valuable lesson for improving the long-term care services in this country can be learned from experiences in several other countries. A significant issue is the relationship between health care and social care systems, and whether or not this can be made harmonious: "In the United States, although not in many European nations, institutional care of the elderly is conceived of and financed as a health service rather than a social service even though institutional placements provide a complete social context for an individual and obviously constitutes a rather dramatic social intervention" (Kane and Kane 1978).

Another important factor is the sponsorship and control of and payment for long-term care services: "In European countries, where long-term care is well developed, it is usually under government sponsorship; the most common pattern is that institutional care is under local government control with conformity to national guidelines" (Kane and Kane 1978). Where nursing homes are well-established in European countries, they are better funded than in the United States. Where, in contrast, there are mixed sponsorships and varied sources of regulation, control is primarily the function of the federal government, and long-term care services are generally underfunded.

Experiences in European countries have demonstrated that programs cannot be substituted for one another; both home care services and institutional care are needed to provide the range of options important to developing long-term care programs.

While it seems appropriate to stress the social care organization as the primary method of structuring long-term care, it is essential that the medical care provider be an active partner in the health care team. In Great Britain, geriatrics is a well-developed and growing medical specialty. In addition, the family care practitioner provides the first line of medical care. This is not to say that a simple resolution of our problems would be to adopt the practices of European countries. While we can learn much from other practices, our basic need is to define our own problems and find solutions to them. Furthermore, the absence of policy and commitment creates many of our problems. According to Kane and Kane (1978), "we have addressed our willingness to support elderly citizens more by incremental default than by positive programs designed to provide comfort and dignity. To some observers, it may appear that our efforts on behalf of those in the unproductive phases of their life cycle have been designed to protect the more productive elements of society from the burdens of providing direct care."

Consistent with the emphasis on vigorous response to the needs of those who are currently chronically ill is the rationale that research into more efficient and effective service modalities, and demonstrations of them, is appropriate and deserves public support. We can argue that the physical, emotional, and social needs of the chronically ill are as great as those of the millions who are either institutionalized or severely restricted in their own homes, and deserve the primary attention of a humane society. After all, these are our progenitors, who provided for us in our early years. We owe them our support because of the severe limitations of their current status. Their need for our human compassion could not be greater.

We can argue also that their very presence as dependent, disabled older people is a product of our society's successful battle with some of the acute illnesses, and that the large numbers of chronically ill are testimony to the crisis we have created. The issues of age-related physiological decrements have been intensified by our medical achievements, and remain "unfinished business." We have been successful in extending the life expectancy for many, but have not adequately addressed some of the increased problems related to the quality of the additional years granted to these older persons (Engelhardt 1977).

The importance of humanism in health care, the "quality of life" issue, is not confined to the elderly. The remarkable technology of health care and the great successes of modern medicine have also, according to Howard and Derzon, "blinded caregivers and even their patients to a loss that each has sustained amidst the triumphs of medicine—a loss of the humanism that is so integral to the underlying premises of health care." They go on to describe humane care as follows:

> Patients are perceived as unique and irreplaceable whole persons who are inherently worthy of the caregiver's concern. To the extent of their capacity, they share in decisions that affect their care and their relations with providers are egalitarian or reciprocal, not deferential or patronizing. Within the limits imposed by illness and rules that protect society, recipients of humanized care function as autonomous persons who have a right to control their own destinies. Moreover, they are treated with empathy and warmth by their caregivers.

The same standards of humanized care must also be applied to the care providers. Providers who are exploited or dehumanized will find it difficult to treat their patients humanistically, especially those patients who are chronically ill. Concern for costs in health care, expansion of medical technology, and shortages at key staff positions have made it harder for health care providers to concentrate on the caring part of their functions. Quality of life issues, the increasing numbers of chronically ill needing health services, and the emergence of hospice care have ushered in a new era of humanistic health care. All who are involved in health care, providers and recipients alike, will benefit from this new humanism, which has been accompanied by greater concern for developing supportive environments and life-styles compatible with the maintenance of good health. Preventive care practices, with individuals assuming greater responsibility for their own health, is part of this evolution. A recent report by the United States Surgeon General on health, prevention, and disease listed goals for improvement of health of all age sectors in our society. Specific goals of those over sixty-five were: "A major improvement in health, mobility, and independence for older people, to be achieved largely by reducing by 20 percent the average number of days of illness among this age group" (Public Health Reports 1979).

Equally ambitious but realizable goals are set forth for the full range of age categories. In the sense that these represent a goal of the federal government, they are in conflict with the public policy of Medicare, which attempts to discourage early use of health care services. In addition to its built-in deductible and coinsurance charges, Medicare will not pay for preventive services. As a sick care service only, Medicare cannot help older people reduce the number of days of illness by reimbursing them for the cost of preventive measures. The number of days of illness can be reduced through early health care intervention, a practice that should be supported through a health care payment program for the elderly. The fact that so many older Americans are also poor makes this an especially important issue. Additionally, "days of illness" generally refers to the acute episode of any illness. The number of these days could often be reduced by taking advantage of the skills of appropriate diagnosis and initiating early intervention of the therapeutic regime prescribed. The millions of older people living alone without substantial health support services available to them may have no way to pursue a course of therapy that will lead to prompt recuperation. Again, the health care payment policies of the federal government are not supportive of the intensive home care services that could be most helpful to isolated older people.

Furthermore, reducing days of chronic illness is not a realizable goal because chronic illnesses, if not cured, are generally terminated by death. Once again, the goal of reducing the average number of days of illness, although admirable, is not related to chronic illness, the major problem of older people. Appropriate reduction in disabling illnesses and accidents among the younger age cohorts may be one way of achieving better health for older people. Changing life-styles will probably lead to healthier older people, and need to be encouraged by vigilant government agencies identifying those elements of societal life that may have a deleterious impact on health and acting to overcome them. Massive education and enforcement campaigns are needed to support government action to protect all age groups from the disease-spreading vectors, environmental contaminants, safety hazards, or merely qualities of our life-style that may be injurious to our health.

We have almost been led to believe that those over seventy-five, the group that Neugarten calls the old-old, are destined to face intractable problems of ill health and dependency because of the clear association of this age group with the ever-increasing incidence of disabling chronic illness. We especially project increases in incontinence, mental impairment, cardiovascular disease, cancer, cerebral accidents, failing eyesight, and accidental injuries such as fractured hips. We expect that the incidence of hospitalization, prolonged illness, institutionalization, and poverty are all age-related products of the increase in life expectancy, and we respond with efforts to offset the ill effects of this increased period of life with rehabilitative, restorative, and other ameliorative interventions. But as Hayflick points out in his illustration (1977) of the response of the National Foundation for Infantile Paralysis to polio in the 1940s and 1950s: "Had the Foundation decided at that time to invest all or most of its resources in the perfection of better iron lungs, we would probably have today the best designed, best automated, and exquisitely comfortable iron lung for tens of thousands of current polio victims. Instead, the Foundation made the decision that a substantial portion of its resources should be invested in the basic research necessary to understand and control the disease. The outcome, of course, is familiar to us all."

While substantially improved resources for the chronically ill are still required, he goes on: "One goal appears to be wholly desirable and even attainable as a short-range objective. This is simply to reduce the physiological decrements associated with biological aging so that vigorous, productive nondependent lives would be led up until the mean maximum lifespan of, say, one hundred years. Implicit in this notion is that the quality of life is more important than its quantity."

For the chronically ill, the prolongation of life is of necessity a prolongation of the period of pain and dependency. The successful introduction of hospice care into programs provided for patients with terminal illness illustrates the readiness of society to reject the notion of value in the prolongation of life without proper regard for the quality of life. Hospice care rejects the artificial sustenance of life that cannot be lived with dignity.

Many of us would subscribe to what Hayflick outlines as the ideal shape of a human life: that we could realize the ultimate rectangular life expectancy curve in which all causes of death resulting from disease and accidents are totally eliminated, where the decrements of chronic illnesses no longer existed, where people would live out their lives free from the fear of the effects of chronic illness but assured that they would die on the eve of their hundredth birthdays.

# Appendix

# A

## Significant Legislation Related to Long-Term Care

1935    Passage of the Social Security Act. Established the first nationwide institutional structure to assist older Americans.

1946    Hill-Burton Program instituted (Public Law 79-482, Medical Facilities Survey and Construction Act). Provided funds for the construction and equipping of nursing homes and hospitals. Introduced planning for health care facilities.

1948    Task force on aging set up by the Federal Security Agency (predecessor of the Department of Health, Education, and Welfare).

1950    First National Conference on Aging.

1953    Federal aid authorized for the cost of assistance paid to indigent persons in private institutions.

1956    Housing Act of 1956 passed (Public Law 84-1020), including Section 404 on housing for the elderly. Public housing legislation modified to accommodate the special problems of the elderly.

1958    Small Business Administration authorized through the Small Business Act and the Small Business Investment Act to provide loans to nursing homes.

1959    National Housing Act amended to provide for mortgage insurance to private lenders to facilitate construction or rehabilitation of proprietary and nonprofit nursing homes.

1960    Passage of the Federal Assistance for the Aged Act, providing a broad-based program of federal financial assistance to the states to furnish care for the indigent and the medically indigent in a wide variety of institutional and noninstitutional programs.

1961    White House Conference on Aging.

1965    Title XVIII of the Social Security Act (Medicare) passed, providing for payment of posthospital care in nursing care facilities.

Title XIX, the Medical Assistance title, passed, requiring states to include inpatient and outpatient hospital services, laboratory and X-ray services, skilled nursing-home care, and physicians' services in their vendor payment programs.

Older Americans Act passed, setting forth congressional policy concerning older Americans and the responsibility of the state and federal governments, and providing for demonstration projects, research, and training programs.

1969    Area wide model projects authorized in amendments to the Older Americans Act.

1971    White House Conference on Aging.

1972    Nutrition programs for the aged approved as amendments to the Older Americans Act.

Supplementary Security Income (SSI) program passed as an amendment to the Social Security Act of 1935.

1973    Federal Council on Aging established by amendments to the Older Americans Act.

Federal Health Maintenance Organization Act passed, setting the stage for a new payment mechanism for health care.

1974    Passage of the National Health Planning and Resources Development Act, combining and redirecting the efforts of a number of federally supported state and local agencies (i.e., the Hill-Burton Program begun in 1946), the Regional Medical Program enacted in 1965, and the Comprehensive Health Planning Program of 1966. The new act established the Health Systems Agencies.

Patient's Bill of Rights introduced to protect the rights of nursing home patients.

Passage of the Title XX Amendments to the Social Security Act of 1935, providing grants to states to provide social services, many of which are for the elderly.

1975    Creation of the National Institute on Aging.

1977    Legislation passed in California mandating payment for adult day care through Title XIX.

1978    Passage of comprehensive Older Americans Act amendments, reinforcing support for senior centers and coordination of programs in long-term care.

Department of Housing and Urban Development authorized by the Congregate Housing Services Program to enter into contracts with local public housing agencies and with nonprofit corporations to provide congregate services.

Channeling Grants Program initiated to support the development of comprehensive, coordinated systems of community long-term care.

1980    Funding initiated a series of Long-Term Care Gerontology Centers based in university settings throughout the country.

1981    White House Conference on Aging.

# Appendix
# B

## Significant Health Care Program Development Dates in the United States

1751    Pennsylvania Hospital founded—first hospital in the United States.

1796    Beginning of home health care.

1842    First Catholic Home for the Aged.

1855    First Jewish Home for the Aged.

1885    First voluntary home health agency established, in Buffalo, New York.

1903    "Gerontology" first used to describe the study of senescence.

1909    "Geriatrics" coined as name for the study of clinical aspects of aging.

1927    American Association for Old Age Security founded. (Became American Association for Social Security in 1933.)

1940    Penicillin and other antibiotics introduced.

1943    First senior center, the William Hodson Community Center, opened in New York City.

1947    Hospital-based home health care program begun by Montefiore Hospital in New York City.

1951    Centralized intake initiated in Chicago.

1961    American Association of Homes for the Aged organized.

1965    First private day care program opened, in Beverly Hills, California.

1967    First network of day care programs developed, in Tucson, Arizona.

1970    National Institute of Senior Centers organized by the National Council on the Aging.

National Association of Home Health Agencies organized.

Monroe County Demonstration Program initiated. Special service for diagnosis, evaluation, and placement of the chronically ill and elderly.

1972    Area wide model project on alternatives to institutional care developed in Tucson, Arizona.

1974    American Health Care Association organized.

1977    Full service inpatient and home care program opened by Hillhaven Hospice.

# References

"Access." New York: Monroe County Long Term Care Program, Inc., 1979.

Achenbaum, W. A. *Old Age in the New Land: The American Experience from 1790.* Baltimore, Md.: Johns Hopkins University Press, 1978.

Ainsworth, T. H. *Quality Assurance in Long Term Care.* Germantown, Md.: Aspen Systems Corp., 1977.

Altieri, A. J.; M. E. Sedutto; H. M. Feder; and M. S. Weissman. "Developing Quality Long Term Care." *Geriatrics* 32, no. 7 (1977): 126–42.

Anderson, O. "Reflections on the Sick Aged and Helping Systems." In *Social Policy, Social Ethics and the Aging Society,* ed. B. Neugarten and R. Havighurst, pp. 89–96. Washington, D.C.: National Science Foundation, 1976.

Anderson, W. F. "Achievements in Geriatric Medicine." In *Recent Advances in Gerontology.* Amsterdam, The Netherlands: Excerpta Medica, 1979.

Barney, J. "The Prerogative of Choice in Long Term Care." *Gerontologist* 17, no. 4 (1977): 309–14.

Beattie, W. "Aging and the Social Services." In *Handbook of Aging and the Social Services,* ed. R. H. Binstock and E. Shanas. New York: Van Nostrand Reinhold, 1976.

Bell, W. G. "Community Care for the Elderly: An Alternative to Institutionalization." *Gerontologist* 13, no. 3 (1973): 349–54.

Bengston, V. L. "The Aged and Their Families: Constructs and Measurements of Intergenerational Relationships." *Recent Advances in Gerontology.* Amsterdam, The Netherlands: Excerpta Medica, 1979.

Bergman, S. "The Future of Human Welfare of the Aged." *Recent Advances in Gerontology.* Amsterdam, The Netherlands: Excerpta Medica, 1979.

Binstock, R. H., and M. A. Levin. "The Political Dilemmas of Intervention Policies." In *Handbook of Aging and the Social Sciences,* ed. R. H. Binstock and E. Shanas. New York: Van Nostrand Reinhold Co., 1976.

Boynton, R. *The Housing of Independent Elderly.* Occasional Papers in Housing and Community Affairs, vol. 1. Washington, D.C.: U.S. Department of Housing and Urban Development, 1978.

Brickner, P. W. "Health Care Services for Homebound Aged Maintain Independence, Limit Costs." *Hospital Progress* 61, no. 9 (1980): 56–9.

———. *Home Health Care for the Aged.* New York: Appleton-Century-Crofts, 1978.

Brody, E. M. *Long Term Care of Older People.* New York: Human Science Press, 1977.

Brody, S. J.; S. W. Poulshock; and C. F. Masciocchi. "The Family Caring Unit: A Major Consideration in the Long Term Support System." *Gerontologist* 18, no. 6 (1978): 556–61.

Brook, R. H. "Quality, Can We Measure It?" *New England Journal of Medicine,* 296 (June 1977): 197.

Brotman, H. B. "The Aging of America: A Demographic Profile." In *The Economics of Aging. National Journal Issues Book.* Washington, D.C.: Government Research Corporation, 1978.

Brown, E. L. *Newer Dimensions of Patient Care.* New York: Russell Sage Foundation, 1961.

Butler, R. M. Quoted in *Old Age in the New Land,* ed. W. A. Achenbaum. Baltimore, Md.: Johns Hopkins University Press, 1978. Butler is merely quoted in the book.

Callihan, J. J. "The Organization of Long Term Care System and the Potential For a Single Agency Option." Mimeographed. Waltham, Mass.: Brandeis University, 1979.

Campbell, M. "Study of the Attitudes of Nursing Personnel Towards the Geriatric Patient." *Nursing Research* 20, no. 2 (1971): 147–51.

Carp, F. "The Concept and Role of Congregate Housing for Older People." *Congregate Housing for Older People.* Washington, D.C.: U.S. Dept. of Health, Education, and Welfare, 1977.

Cherkasky, M. "The Montefiore Hospital Home Care Program." *American Journal of Public Health* 39 (February 1949): 163–66.

Cohen, E. "An Overview of Long Term Care Facilities." In *A Social Work Guide for Long Term Care Facilities,* ed. E. Brody. Washington, D.C.: National Institute of Mental Health, 1977.

Comptroller General of the United States. "Home Health—The Need for a National Policy to Better Provide for the Elderly." Washington, D.C.: General Accounting Office, December 1977.

Cottrell, F. "Overview of Ethical Issues." In *Ethical Considerations in Long Term Care,* ed. W. E. Winston and W. J. E. Wilson. St. Petersburg, Fla.: Eckerd Gerontology Center, 1977.

Crowley, D., and D. Cloud. "Aging Advocacy at the National Level." *Aging.* U.S. Dept. of Health, Education, and Welfare, nos. 297–98 (July-August 1979): 13–17.

Cyrus-Lutz, C., and C. Gaitz. "Psychiatrists' Attitudes Towards the Aged and Aging." *Gerontologist* 12, no. 2 (Summer 1972): 163–67.

Davis, J., and M. Gibbin. "An Areawide Examination of Nursing Home Use, Misuse, and Nonuse." *American Journal of Public Health* 61, no. 6 (June 1971), 1146–55.

Deuschle, J. M.; D. N. Logsdon; W. Sollecito; W. Stahl; H. Smith; M. Sonnenshein; and M. Kreitzer. "Implementation of a Peer Review System for Ambulatory Care." *Public Health Reports* 93, no. 3 (May-June 1978): 258–67.

Dieck, M. "Residential and Community Provisions for the Frail Elderly in Germany: Current Issues and Their History." *Gerontologist* 20, no. 3 (June 1980): 260–72.

Dittman, D. A., and J. A. Peters. "PSRO and HSA, A Federal System of Local Health Care Regulation." *Community Medicine* 42, no. 11 (November 1978): 725–31.

Doherty, N., and B. Hicks. "Cost Effectiveness Analysis and Alternative Health Care Programs for the Elderly." *Health Services Research* 12 (Summer 1977): 190–203.

Donahue, W.; M. Thompson; and D. Curren, eds. *Congregate Housing For Older People.* Washington, D.C.: HEW, Administration on Aging, 1977.

Dunlop, B. D. "Expanded Home-Based Care for the Impaired Elderly: Solution or Pipe Dream." *American Journal of Public Health* 70, no. 5 (May 1980): 514–19.

Englehardt, H. "Treating Aging: Restructuring the Human Condition." In *Extending the Human Life Span: Social Policy and Social Ethics.* ed. B. Neugarten and R. Havighurst. Chicago: University of Chicago Press, 1977.

Ernst, M., and H. Shore. *Sensitizing People to the Process of Aging.* Dallas: Dallas Geriatric Research Institute, 1975.

Estes, C. L. *The Aging Enterprise.* San Francisco: Jossey-Bass, 1979.

Federal Council on the Aging. *Public Policy and the Frail Elderly.* Washington, D.C.: HEW, 1978.

Feldman, J.; R. Burke; and J. Schwarzmann. "Analysis of the Training of Unlicensed Long Term Care Personnel." *The Journal of Long Term Care Administration* 6, no. 2 (Summer 1978): 1–11.

Fischer, D. H. *Growing Old in America.* New York: Oxford University Press, 1978.

Fox, P. D., and S. B. Clauser. "Trends in Nursing Home Expenditures: Implications for Aging Policy." *Health Care Financing Review* 2, no. 2 (Fall 1980): 65–70.

Freeman, J. *Aging: Its History and Literature.* New York: Human Sciences Press, 1979.

Friedman, E. "The Impact of Aging in the Social Structure." In *Handbook of Social Gerontology.* ed. C. Tibbits. Chicago: The University of Chicago Press, 1960.

Fromm, E. *The Art of Loving.* New York: Bantam Books, 1956.

Gadow, S. "Medicine, Ethics, and the Elderly." *Gerontologist* 20, no. 6 (1980): 680–85.

Geiger, D. "Note: How Future Professionals View the Elderly: A Comparative Analysis of Social Work, Law, and Medical Students' Perceptions." *Gerontologist* 18, no. 6 (1978): 591–94.

Gibson, R. M. "The Newcastle Experience." *Recent Advances in Gerontology.* Amsterdam, The Netherlands. Excerpta Medica, 1979.

Gold, J., and S. Kaufman. "Development of Care of Elderly: Tracing the History of Institutional Facilities." *Gerontologist* 10, no. 4 (Winter 1970): 262–74.

Greenberg, J. "The Cost of In-Home Services." In *A Planning Study of Services to Non-Institutional Older Persons in Minnesota,* ed. N. Anderson. St. Paul: Governor's Citizens Council on Aging, 1974.

Gruber, H. "Geriatrics—Physician Attitudes and Medical School Training." *American Geriatrics Society Conference on Geriatric Education* 25, no. 11 (1977): 494–96.

Grunow, D. "Sozialstationen: A New Model for Home Delivery of Care and Service." *Gerontologist* 20, no. 3 (1980): 308–17.

Gutowski, M. F. "Integrating Housing and Social Services Activities for the Elderly Household." In *Occasional Papers in Housing and Community Affairs: The Housing of Independent Elderly.* Washington, D.C.: HUD vol. 1 (1978): 110–30.

Hayflick, L. "Perspectives on Human Longevity." In *Extending the Human Life Span: Social Policy and Social Ethics.* eds. B. Neugarten and R. Havighurst. Chicago: University of Chicago Press, 1977.

Health Care Financing Administration. *Directory of Adult Day Care Centers.* Rockville, Md.: HEW, 1978.

————. *Long Term Care: Background and Future Directions.* Washington, D.C.: HEW, 1981.

Hendricks, J., and C. D. Hendricks. *Aging in Mass Society.* Cambridge, Mass.: Winthrop, 1981.

Hinkley, N. "Staff Development: A Frill, A Requirement, or A Necessity?" *Journal of Long Term Care Administration* 6, no. 2 (Summer 1978): 12–19.

Howard, J., and R. Derzon. "Prospects for Humane Care Are Hopeful." *Hospitals* 53, no. 22 (November 1979): 76–9.

Human, J. "Normative Planning for a Better Long Term Care System." *American Journal of Health Planning* 1, no. 2 (October 1976): 43–7.

Iglehart, J. "The Cost of Keeping the Elderly Well." In *The Economics of Aging, A National Journal Issue Book.* Washington, D.C.: Government Research Corp., 1978.

Institute of Medicine. *Aging and Medical Education.* Washington, D.C.: National Academy of Sciences, 1978.

Ishizaki, B.; L. Gottesman; and S. MacBride. "Determinants of Model Choice for Service Management System." *Gerontologist* 19, no. 4 (1979): 376–85.

Joe, T., and Meltzer, Judith. "Policies and Strategies for Long-Term Care," Health Policy Program School of Medicine, University of California, San Francisco, CA, May 14, 1976.

Jones, E. W.; P. M. Denson; B. J. McNitt. *Assessing the Quality of Long Term Care.* Washington, D.C.: HEW, 1978.

Kahn, A. J., and S. B. Kammerman. *Not for the Poor Alone.* Philadelphia: Temple University Press, 1976.

Kammerman, S. B., and A. J. Kahn. *Social Services in the United States.* Philadelphia: Temple University Press, 1976.

Kane, R. L., and R. A. Kane. "Alternatives to Institutional Care of the Elderly: Beyond the Dichotomy." *Gerontologist* 20, no. 3 (1980 a): 249–59.

————. "Care of the Aged: Old Problems in Need of New Solutions." *Science* 200 (26 May 1978): 913–19.

————. "Long-Term Care: Can Our Society Meet the Needs of Its Elderly?" *Annual Review Public Health* 1 (1980 b): 227–53.

————. *Long Term Care in Six Countries.* Washington, D.C.: HEW, NIH, 1976.

Kaplan, J. "An Editorial: Alternative to Nursing Home Care: Fact or Fiction." *Gerontologist* 12, no. 2 (1972): 114.

Kastenbaum, R. "The Reluctant Therapist." *Geriatrics* 18 (April 1963): 296–301.

Kastenbaum, R., and S. E. Candy. "The 4% Fallacy: A Methodological and Empirical Critique of Extended Care Facility Population Statistics." *International Journal of Aging and Human Development* 4, no. 1 (1973): 15–21.

Katzen, F. "The Older Person Experiences a Crisis: The Family Agency and the Alternatives to Institutional Care." In *Geriatric Institutional Management,* ed. M. Leeds and H. Shore. New York: G. P. Putnam's Sons, 1964, pp. 51–6.

Kaufman, A. "Social Policy and Long-Term Care of the Aged." *Social Work* 25, no. 2 (March 1980): 133–7.

Kerschner, P. A., and M. Cote. "Deficiencies in Terminology: The Effect on Public Policy." In *Long Term Care of the Aging: A Socially Responsible Approach,* ed. L. W. Wasser. Washington, D.C.: American Association of Homes for the Aging, 1979.

Kistin, H., and R. Morris. "Alternatives to Institutional Care for the Elderly and Disabled." *Gerontologist* 12, no. 2 (Summer 1972): 139–42.

Kleh, J. "When to Institutionalize the Elderly." *Hospital Practice* (February 1977): 121–25.

Koff, T. *Hospice: A Caring Community.* Cambridge, Mass.: Winthrop Publishers, 1980.

Koncelik, J. A. *Designing the Open Nursing Home.* Stroudsburg, Pa.: Dowden, Hutchinson, and Ross, 1976.

Kuperberg, J. R. "Ethics, Accountability and Decision Making." *Journal of Long Term Care Administration* 6, no. 3 (Fall 1978): 25–34.

Lamden, R., and L. Greenstein. "Partnership in Outpatient Day Care." *Hospitals* 49 (16 October 1975): 87–9.

Lawton, M. P. "Institutions and Alternatives for Older People." *Health and Social Work* 3, no. 2 (May 1978): 108–134.

———. "Social Ecology and the Health of Older People." *American Journal of Public Health* 64, no. 3 (March 1974): 257–60.

Lawton, M. P., and E. M. Brody. "Assessment of Older People: Self-Maintaining and Instrumental Activities of Daily Living." *Gerontologist* 9, no. 3 (1969): 179–86.

Lawton, M. P.; R. J. Newcomer; and T. O. Byers. *Community Planning For an Aging Society.* Stroudsburg, Pa.: Dowden, Hutchinson, and Ross, 1976.

Leanse, J. *Directory of Senior Centers and Clubs.* Washington, D.C.: The National Council on Aging, Inc., 1974.

Leanse, J.; M. Tevin; and T. B. Robb. *Senior Center Operation.* Washington, D.C.: National Institute of Senior Centers, 1977.

Leeds, M. "Geriatric Implications of the Medical Revolution." In *Geriatric Instrumental Management.* ed. M. Leeds and H. Shore. New York: G. P. Putnam's Sons, 1964.

Lipman, A. "Impact of Demographic Changes of Family." *Recent Advances in Gerontology.* Amsterdam, The Netherlands: Excerpta Medica, 1979.

Long Term Care: *Background and Future Directions.* Washington, D.C.: HEW, 1981.

Lorenze, E.; C. Hamill; and R. Oliver. "The Day Hospital: An Alternative to Institutional Care." *Journal of the American Geriatrics Society* 22, no. 7 (1974): 316–20.

Lurie, E.; R. Kalish; R. Wexler; and M. L. Ansak. "On Lok Senior Day Health Center." *Gerontologist* 16, no. 1 (1976): 39–46.

Mayeroff, N. *On Caring.* New York: Harper and Row, 1971.

McEvers, B. "Areawide Model Project: Alternatives to Institutional Care." Tucson, Ariz.: Pima Council on Aging, 1976.

Mechanic, D. "Ethics, Justice and Medical Care Systems." *The Annals of the American Academy of Political and Social Science* 437 (May 1978): 74–85.

Mehta, N., and C. Mack. "Day Care Services: An Alternative to Institutional Care." *Journal of the American Geriatrics Society* 23, no. 6 (1975): 280–3.

Miller, D. B.; R. Lowenstein; and R. Winston. "Physicians' Attitudes Towards the Ill Aged and Nursing Homes." *Journal of the American Geriatric Society* 24 (November 1976): 498–504.

Miller, M. C., and R. G. Knapp. *Evaluating the Quality of Care.* Germantown, Maryland: Aspen Systems Corp., 1977.

Monahan, D., and T. Koff. "Report on a Training Grant with The Pima County

(Arizona) Long Term Care System." Tucson, Ariz.: Univ. of Arizona, 1979. Unpublished.

Okazaki, Y. "Aging of the Japanese Population and Its Demographic, Economic, and Social Implications." *Recent Advances in Gerontology.* Amsterdam, The Netherlands: Excerpta Medica, 1979.

Pfeiffer, E. *Multidimensional Assessment of Three Populations of the Elderly.* Durham, North Carolina: Duke University, 1973.

———. "Multidimensional Functional Assessment: Why and How?" Durham, North Carolina: Duke University, 1973.

Philibert, M. "Philosophy of Aging: Implications for Nursing." *Nursing and the Aged.* New York: McGraw Hill, 1976.

Pinker, R. A. "Facing Up to the Eighties: Health and Welfare Needs of British Elderly." *Gerontologist* 20, no. 3 (1980): 273–83.

Professional Standards Review Organization. *PSRO First Annual Report.* Washington, D.C.: Health Care Financing Administration, HEW, April, 1978.

Quinn, J. L. "Triage: Coordinated Home Care for the Elderly." *Nursing Outlook* 23, no. 9 (September 1975): 570–73.

Rakowski, W., and T. Hickey. "Late Life Health Behavior." *Research on Aging* 2, no. 3 (September 1980): pp. 283–308.

Regan, J., and G. Springer. "Protective Services for the Elderly." By the Special Committee on Aging. Washington, D.C.: United States Senate, 1977.

Reich, W. T. "Ethical Issues Related to Research Involving Elderly Subjects." *Gerontologist* 18, no. 4 (1978): 326–37.

Riffle, K. "Rehabilitation: The Evolution of a Concept." *Nursing Clinics of North America* 8, no. 4 (December 1973): 665–71.

Moos, R. H. "Specialized Living Environments for Older People: A Conceptual Framework for Evaluation." *Journal of Social Issues* 36, no. 2 (1980): 75–94.

Morris, R. "The Development of Parallel Services for the Elderly and Disabled." *Gerontologist* 14, no. 1 (February 1974): 14–19.

Moss, F. E., and V. J. Halamandaris. *Too Old, Too Sick, Too Bad.* Germantown, Maryland: Aspen Systems Corp., 1977.

Mote, J. R. "Continuing Education: Enhancing the Quality of Patient Care." *Hospitals* 50, no. 15 (1 August 1976): 175–80.

National Conference on Social Welfare. *The Future of Long Term Care in the United States.* Washington, D.C.: HEW, 1977.

National Council on Aging. *Directory on Aging.* Washington, D.C.: NCOA, 1974.

National League for Nursing. *Directory of Home Health Agencies, Certified As Medicare Providers.* New York: NLN, 1975.

Neuberger, R. L., and K. Loe. *An Army of the Aged.* New York: DaCapo Press, 1973.

Neugarten, B. L. "Age Groups in American Society and the Rise of the Young—Old." *Annals of American Academy of Political and Social Science* (September 1974): 187–8.

Office of Policy, Planning and Evaluation, Medical Services Administration, Social and Rehabilitation Service. *Day Care Services.* Washington, D.C.: HEW, October 1972.

Robb, S. "Attitudes and Intentions of Bacclaureate Nursing Students Toward the Elderly." *Nursing Research* 28, no. 1 (1979): 43–50.

Rossman, I. "Alternatives to Institutional Care." *Bulletin of the New York Academy of Medicine* 49, no. 12 (December 1973): 1084–92.

————. "Options for Care of the Aged Sick." *Hospital Practice* 12, no. 3 (March 1977): 107–16.

Ruchlin, H. "A New Strategy for Regulating Long-Term Care Facilities." *Journal of Health Politics, Policy and Law* 2, no. 2 (Summer 1977): 190–211.

Ryder, C.; P. Stitt; and W. Elkins. "Home Health Services—Past, Present, Future." *American Journal of Public Health* 59, no. 9 (1969): 1720–29.

Schock, S. "The Urgent Need: Education and Training." *Generations* 5, no. 3 (Spring 1981): 26–41.

Scitovsky, A. A., and N. M. Snyder. *Medical Care Use by a Group of Fully Insured Aged.* Washington, D.C.: National Center for Health Services Research, 1975.

Shanas, E. "Social Myth as Hypothesis: The Case of the Family Relations of Old People." *Gerontologist* 19, no. 1 (1979): 3–9. a

————. "The Family as a Social Support System in Old Age." *Gerontologist* 19, no. 2 (1979): 169–74. b

————. "Measuring the Home Health Needs of the Aged in Five Countries." *Journal of Gerontology* 26, no. 1 (1971): 37–40.

————. *Old People in Three Industrial Societies.* New York: Atherton Press, 1968.

Sherwood, S. "Long-Term Care: Issues, Perspectives and Directions." In *Long Term Care: A Handbook for Researchers, Planners, and Providers.* ed. S. Sherwood. New York: Spectrum Publications, 1975.

Sherwood, S.; J. Morris; and E. Barnhart. "Developing a System for Assigning Individuals Into an Appropriate Residential Setting." *Journal of Gerontology* 30, no. 3 (1975): 331–42.

Shore, H. "What's New About Alternatives?" *Gerontologist* 14, no. 1 (February 1974): 6–11.

Sicker, M. "The AoA Advocacy Assistance Program: Origins and Directions." *Aging.* U.S. Dept. of Health, Education, and Welfare, nos. 297–98 (July-August 1979): 18–21.

Smith, K. F., and V. L. Bengtson. "Positive Consequences of Institutionalization: Solidarity Between Elderly and Their Middle-Aged Children." *Gerontologist* 19, no. 5 (1979): 438–47.

Snyder, J. D., and R. Engleman. "PSRO Program Casts an Eye on Long Term Care." *Geriatrics* 32, no. 1 (January 1977): 118–24.

Solomon, K., and R. Vickers. "Attitudes of Health Workers Towards Old People." Journal of the American Geriatrics Society 27, no. 4 (1979): 186–191.

Solomon, R. "Aging Individuals in Long Term Care Need Choice and Autonomy." *Generations* 5, no. 3 (Spring 1981): 32–8.

Spence, D.; E. Feigenbaum; F. Fitzgerald; and J. Roth. "Medical Student Attitudes Towards the Geriatric Patient." *Journal of American Geriatrics Society* 16, no. 9 (1968): 976–83.

State Communities Aid Association. *Report of Arden House Institute on Continuity of Long Term Care.* New York: State Communities Aid Association, 1977.

Steinfeld, J. "Rehabilitation Medicine: A Changing Challenge in a Changing Society." *Archives of Physical Medicine and Rehabilitation* 53, no. 1 (January 1972): 4–9.

Stewart, J. E. *Home Health Care.* St. Louis: C. V. Mosby, 1979.

Tibbits, C. "Introduction." In *Ethical Considerations on Long Term Care,* ed. W. E. Winston and A. J. E. Wilson. St. Petersburg, Fla.: Eckerd College Gerontology Center, 1977.

Tomlinson, K. R.; B. Trager; and B. Cohen. "Directions for Policy-Related Long Term Care Research." Unpublished. Berkeley, Calif.: University of California School of Public Health, 1976.

Townsend, P. "The Effects of Family Structure on the Likelihood of Admission to an Institution in Old Age: The Application of a General Theory." In *Social Structure and the Family,* ed. E. Shanas and G. F. Streib. Englewood Cliffs, N.J.: Prentice-Hall, 1965.

Trager, B. Adult Day Health Care—A Conference Report. Tucson: University of Arizona, 1979.

————. "Home Health Services in the United States: A Report to the Special Committee on Aging." United States Senate, 1972. Unpublished.

U.S. Dept. of Health, Education, and Welfare. *An Overview of Nursing Home Characteristics: Provisional Data from the 1977 National Nursing Survey.* Washington, D.C., 1978.

————. *Comprehensive Older Americans Act Amendments of 1978.* Washington, D.C.: HEW, 1978.

————. "Home Care for Persons Fifty-five Years and Over: United States, July 1965-June 1968." In *Vital and Health Statistics Series* 10, no. 73 (1972). National Center for Health Statistics.

————. "Prevention, A Challenge to the Nation." *Public Health Reports* 94, no. 5 (1979): 483–5.

————. Public Health Service. *Vital and Health Statistics of the National Center for Health Statistics,* no. 35 (September 6, 1978).

U.S. Dept. of Housing and Urban Development. *Evaluation of Effectiveness of Congregate Housing for the Elderly.* Washington, D.C.: HUD, 1976.

U.S. Dept. of Public Health and Welfare. *Title XX Grants to States for Services.* Code: 42:1397.

U.S. National Committee on Vital and Health Statistics. *Long Term Care: Minimum Data Set.* Washington, D.C.: HEW, 1978.

Volk, L.; J. B. Hutchins; and J. S. Doremus. "A National Cost-Containment Strategy for Long Term Care." *Public Administration Review* 40, no. 5 (September/October 1980): 747–79.

Weg, R. *Nutrition and the Later Years.* Los Angeles: University of Southern California Press, 1978.

Weissert, W.; T. Wan; B. Livieratos; and S. Katz. "Effects and Costs of Day Care Services for the Chronically Ill." *Medical Care* 18, no. 6 (June 1980): 567–84.

Welfield, I., and R. Struyk. *Housing Options for the Elderly.* Occasional Papers in Housing and Community Affairs, vol. 3. Washington, D.C.: HUD, 1978.

White House Conference on Families. *Listening to America's Families: Action For the '80s.* Washington, D.C.: HEW, 1980.

Wilson, S. H. "Nursing Home Patients' Rights, Are They Enforceable?" *Gerontologist* 18, no. 3 (1978): 255–61.

Winn, S., and K. M. McCaffree. "Issues Involved in the Development of a Prepaid Capitation Plan for Long Term Care Services." *Gerontologist* 19, no. 2 (1979): 184–90.

York, J. L., and R. J. Calsyn. "Family Involvement in Nursing Homes." *Gerontologist* 17, no. 6 (1977): 500–5.

# Index

Nursing Homes. *See also* Institutional care
demographics, 15, 19
Nutrition services, 49–50
funding, 50
programs, 49–50

Okazaki, Y., 14
Older Americans Act, 4–5, 18, 28–29, 48, 50–52. *See also* Title III—Title XX
amendments (1971), 51
amendments (1972), 50
amendments (1973), 50
amendments (1978), 28–29, 48

Pfeiffer, E., 75
Philabert, M., 104
Pima County, 51
Pinker, R., 14
Poor laws, 35, 38
Professional Standards Review Organization (PSRO), 87, 112
Protective services, 89–90
definition of, 90
Public agencies, 27
Public Health Service, 83
Public information, 72–73
Public policy issues, 28–31, 54, 110–111
funding, 29
quality, 30
research, 31
response to, 31
right to care, 28, 30

Quality care, evaluation of, 111–120
area agency on aging, 115
case management, 118
ethics, 113
financing, 118
Health Systems Agency, 115–116
licensing, 119
patient assessment, 118
patient rights, 114–115
peer review, 117
professional organizations, 117
research, 119
staff availability, 117–118

Rakowski, W., 16
Regan, J., 89, 90
Reich, W., 119
Reimbursement, 23. *See also* Funding; Medicare; Medicaid
Relocation, 24
Riffle, K., 41
Robb, S., 98
Rossman, I., 25
Ruchlin, H., 119
Rush, B., 34
Ryder, C., 44

Schock, S., 96
Service centers, 47–48
definition of, 47
programs, 47–48
Services, 17, 110–113. *See also* Long-term care
distribution of, 110–111
effectiveness of, 112–113
support for family, 17
Services system, 25, 29, 38, 59–65. *See also* Long-term care
comprehensive, 29
entry into, 25
models, 59–65
services, list of, 60–61, 63
Shanas, E., 6, 7, 12, 13, 14, 20
Sherwood, S., 2, 24
Shore, H., 20, 56
Sicker, M., 91, 92
Smith, K., 17
Snyder, J., 116
Social Security Act, 5, 8. *See also* Title programs
Social Security System, history of, 35–36
Solomon, K., 98, 103, 104
Spence, D., 97
Staff development, 100–107
education and training, 102–103
hiring, 100–101
incentives, 101
mobility, 100
nurturing, 105–106
State Communities Aid Association, 38
Stewart, J., 42